Kathryn I. Moghadas, RN, CLRM, CHBC, CHCC, CPC

Tools for an Efficient Medical Practice

Forms, Templates, and Checklists

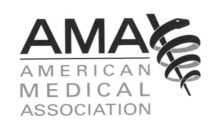

AMA
AMERICAN
MEDICAL
ASSOCIATION

Executive Vice President, Chief Executive Officer: Michael D. Maves, MD, MBA
Chief Operating Officer: Bernard L. Hengesbaugh
Senior Vice President, Publishing and Business Services: Robert A. Musacchio, PhD
Vice President and General Manager, Publishing: Frank J. Krause
Publisher, Physician Practice Solutions: Jay T. Ahlman
Vice President, Business Operations: Vanessa Hayden
Senior Acquisitions Editor: Marsha Mildred
Director, Production and Manufacturing: Jean Roberts
Manager, Developmental Editing: Nancy C. Baker
Developmental Editor: Rebecca Luttrell
Director, Business Marketing and Communication: Pam Palmersheim
Director, Sales and Strategic Partnerships: J. D. Kinney
Senior Production Specialist: Boon Ai Tan
Senior Print Production Specialist: Ronnie Summers
Marketing Manager: Leigh Adams

Internet address: www.ama-assn.org

The authors, editors, and publisher of this work have checked with sources believed to be reliable in their efforts to confirm the accuracy and completeness of the information presented herein and that the information is in accordance with the standard practices accepted at the time of publication. However, neither the authors nor the publisher nor any party involved in the creation and publication of this work warrant that the information is in every respect accurate and complete, and they are not responsible for any errors or omissions or for any consequences from application of the information in this book.

Additional copies of this book may be ordered by calling 800 621-8335 or from the secure AMA web site at www.amabookstore.com. Refer to product number OP127108

ISBN 978-1-60359-000-6
BP22:08-P-033:09/08

Library of Congress Cataloging-in-Publication Data

Moghadas, Kathryn I.
 Tools for an efficient medical practice : forms, templates, and checklists / Kathryn I. Moghadas.
   p. ; cm.
 ISBN 978-1-60359-000-6
 1. Medicine--Practice--Management. 2. Medical offices--Management--Forms. I. American Medical Association. II. Title.

 [DNLM: 1. Practice Management, Medical--Forms. 2. Personnel Management--Forms. W 80 M696m 2009]

 R728.M636 2009
 610.68--dc22

                    2008030838

CONTENTS

CD-ROM (containing all forms, templates, and checklists)

5   OSHA   175

6   CLIA   227

7   Health Insurance Portability and Accountability Act   247

8   Quality Improvement and Risk Management   295

Thank you, Chris Gropp. Your diligence, brilliance, dedication to the project, and general DNA made this book's completion possible. These forms or, actually, their predecessors originated from many sources over the years. John S. Bubula, MBA, CPA, who was chairman of the members services committee of the now-defunct Society of Medical Dental Management Consultants worked diligently, tasking many of us members to submit forms for use by all of us. My thanks go to him for his tireless work that allowed me to take some of those original forms and update them for use today. In addition, the members of the National Society of Certified Healthcare Business Consultants, as well as others, helped supply the forms, templates, and checklist over the years that we have all reinvented to our specific practices. In addition, the AMA released a series of practice support manuals through their Private Advocacy Group, which had some useful templates that they have shared with me in the writing of this book.

Along the way during the development of the book, many individuals were around and supportive, and what a blessing they all are. My gratitude to all of them is hopefully apparent every time I see them. Also, I would like to express gratitude to my Savior Jesus Christ.

My family, Ron and Sarah, continue to provide the stability and sanity necessary to launch another book project. We all know this is not my great American novel; however, to see how proud Ron is, when he is bragging on me, one might get confused. Sarah, who is now 14, has reduced it all into the simple language of, "My mom teaches doctors how to run their business." Our family may be small in numbers, but we are powerful trio. Add Stormy, the dingo dog, to the mix, and we are the mighty. Life cannot get more simple than that. Thank you to everyone who buys the book and those of you who support the process. The highest compliment you can give is to use the book to make your life and the lives of your patients better.

ABOUT THE AUTHOR

Kathryn I. Moghadas is the founder of Associated Healthcare Advisors, Inc., a provider of compliance, risk management, and operational support services for small organizations. Ms Moghadas has been a health care consultant and educator since 1984. Trained as a nurse and risk manager, she is certified in both those disciplines. She also is a certified compliance specialist, certified health care business consultant, and certified professional coder. TopCat, her continuing education school, is licensed for nurses, medical case managers, and insurance adjusters in 38 states.

Ms Moghadas graduated from the George Mason University and Prince Georges College. She is certified in medical office business consulting through the National Society of Certified Healthcare Business Consultants, compliance through Healthcare Compliance Resources, and risk management through the American Board of Healthcare Risk Management, Inc. Ms Moghadas is a contributing editor to several medical management magazines, including *Medical Economics* and *AMA News*. Ms Moghadas published in 2005 through the AMA, *Managing Your Medical Practice*, and in 2000, Chapter 23 titled "Healthcare Regulatory Compliance" and in 1992, chapter 18 titled "Managing Professional Liability Risk" in AHAB Press's annually updated encyclopedia of *Managing Your Medical Practice*. Ms Moghadas lives in the Orlando area with her husband Ron and daughter Sarah.

chapter 1

Starting a Practice

Starting or joining a medical practice is the second phase of a medical career, following education. The time and multiple details required can be managed and attention focused by using forms, checklists, and templates. The forms, checklists, and templates to assist physicians in starting a new practice are included in this chapter. Using these tools can help prevent physicians from being overwhelmed by the tasks involved in starting a practice and help ensure that all essential steps are taken to set up a successful and effective practice that complies with relevant laws, rules, and regulations. A spreadsheet to help track start-up expenses is also included in the chapter, as is a checklist of business references.

Becoming credentialed by a hospital or an insurance carrier requires the provision of standards documents. The credentialing checklist is designed to help maintain order and completeness as the required documents are obtained and collated. The speed of credentialing depends on many factors not within the control of credentialing applicants. However, delays and returns result when the documents provided include inconsistent information and can be avoided or reduced if each individual or entity is identified legally and consistently uses the legal identity in all documents submitted.

Decisions about needed services, supplies, and equipment can require substantial research and comparison of products and vendors. Developing a formal outline, or request for proposals (RFPs), that describes the desired features of services, supplies, and equipment helps clearly identify needs of the practice and provides guidelines to vendors about these needs. An RFP also helps organize information from various vendors so that reliable comparisons can be made more easily and effectively. In addition, RFPs provide a basis for developing a checklist for purchasing equipment and supplies and for stocking and furnishing all rooms in the office to help avoid duplication and costly mistakes.

Other helpful tools in this chapter include practice promotion checklist to provide some structure for promoting the practice and a checklist for the different forms of insurance needed in a medical practice.

Tools for Starting a Practice

Number	Title	Purpose	Notes
01001	Checklist for Credentialing	Many credentialing organizations request the same specific information and documentation that supports the information.	With this form, the user ensures that all names, demographic identifiers, and legal identifier numbers match each other. A complete form should accompany each different person or entitiy seeking credentialing.
01002	Checklist for New Office Supplies	To assist in the purchase of supplies needed to open a practice. The list is a general list of items and should be tailored to suit the specific practice type.	This form can initially be used to establish a budget and later be used to assist in developing a reorder and inventory control list.
01003	Template for a Notice to Patients of No Malpractice Insurance	To notify patients that a physician does not have malpractice insurance	This form is currently required in states that allow physicians to practice without malpractice insurance.
01004	Checklist for Overall Practice Compliance	To assess practice compliance by using this checklist while developing the policies and procedures that address the specific areas on the checklist.	By using this form, the user has the tools to perform a self assessment of their practices compliance program. For assistance in developing the policies and procedures please consult the companion book, *Medical Office Policies and Procedures*.
01005	Checklist for Practice Promotion and Marketing	To ensure that the practice is properly and adequately promoted and marketed	This checklist provides a way to organize your marketing and promotion program.
01006	Form for a Practice Start-up Expenses Spreadsheet	To track practice start-up expenses	A useful form to assist in establishing a start-up budget.
01007	Checklist for Professional Insurance	To assist in identifying different types of insurance needed for a practice	This checklist presents the different types of insurances available to a new practice.
01008	Checklist for Reference Books and Materials	To list a reference library of practice management and billing books	This checklist can be also used to keep track of the materials purchased to support the operations of the practice.
01009	Checklist for Selecting and Equipping a New Practice	To list equipment needed to open a practice	

Number	Title	Purpose	Notes
01010	Template for a Request for Proposal	Major purchases of equipment or services should follow a request for proposal query. With this RFP template, respondents are better equipped to address your specific needs.	This template can serve as a boilerplate request for proposals for services, supplies, and equipment from external service providers. It is used to request specific information from vendors so that comparable types of information are provided. For example, for an office laboratory, the request might identify the anticipated equipment needs and ask vendors to provide the following information for each item: functions available (eg, in a sample analyzer); space, environmental, electrical, and other requirements for effective use of the item; cost; guarantees; availability of service and parts; and lead time needed for delivery and installation.
01011	Checklist for Starting a Practice	To provide a list of steps to open a new practice	This form can also double as a time line for focusing efforts on practice start-ups.
01012	Form for a Board of Directors Listing	To assist in creating the necessary paper trail to assist the accreditation of a practice.	Most accrediting organizations require listing of all the members of the board. This tool can be used when developing an operations manual and for incorporation.
01013	Template for an Organizational Chart	To organizational chart is used to describe the management of your medical practice and the clear lies of authority within your organization. Positions can be used or names of the individuals can be used.	An organizational chart is useful for seeking accreditation and for orientation of physicians and other employees to the practice. The chart should show the relationships of all positions to all other positions.

Credentialing

All documents need to be camera-ready quality or in PDF format. Provide copies only. DO NOT SEND ORIGINALS.

Check if Completed	Credentialing Information Needed	Responsible Party	Date Acquired/Notes
	1. Personal Information		
☐	Legal name, alias	_____	_____
☐	Other name used	_____	_____
☐	Copy of driver's license	_____	_____
☐	Birth: date, state, county, country	_____	_____
☐	Social Security #	_____	_____
☐	Gender	_____	_____
☐	Current address & telephone number	_____	_____
☐	Fingerprint card	_____	_____
☐	NPI #	_____	_____
	2. Professional Identification and Information		
☐	Medical license/state issued	_____	_____
☐	State where physician practices	_____	_____
☐	DEA license number/state or federal issued	_____	_____
☐	Controlled substance license/state issued	_____	_____
☐	Medicare legacy #	_____	_____
☐	Medicaid #	_____	_____
☐	Practice location & telephone number	_____	_____
☐	If using PO Box, PO Box address	_____	_____
☐	Entity or DBA state certificate of status, group entity	_____	_____
☐	SSI proof of TIN #	_____	_____
☐	Occupational permit for city and county	_____	_____
☐	NPI # for entity	_____	_____

Check if Completed	Credentialing Information Needed	Responsible Party	Date Acquired/Notes

2. Professional Identification and Information (continued)

☐ Practice hours of operation _____ _____

☐ CLIA certificate needed for office lab? _____ _____

3. Education and Training

☐ Complete CV with addresses & telephone numbers; education, training, & work histories; description of employment or work gaps of 1 month or longer. _____ _____

☐ Board certification certificate number, date of certification, certification board name, effective date, expiration date. If foreign graduate, copy of ECFMG Certificate. _____ _____

☐ Specialty and secondary specialty _____ _____

4. Insurance Plans

☐ Which carriers, please indicate _____ _____

☐ Get physician numbers from state Medicare carrier _____ _____

☐ Get physician numbers from state Medicaid carrier _____ _____

☐ Get physician numbers from state BC/BS carrier _____ _____

☐ Request fee schedule from Medicare (http://hhs.cms.gov) _____ _____

☐ Enroll in HMOs _____ _____

☐ HMOs/PPOs to participate with contact review _____ _____

☐ IPAs, PHOs, MSOs to participate with
    a. Address
    b. Department
    c. Privilege status
    d. Department directors' names _____ _____

☐ Admitting arrangements _____ _____

☐ Affiliation dates _____ _____

Check if Completed	Credentialing Information Needed	Responsible Party	Amount/Limit and Expiration Date

5. Practice Insurance

☐ Self-insured? _____ _____

☐ Carrier name, address, telephone _____ _____

☐ Copy of insurance face sheet _____ _____

☐ Workers' compensation insurance data _____ _____

6. Reference Information

☐ Three names, addresses, & telephone numbers

1. _____

2. _____

3. _____

7. Bank Information

☐ Voided check with account and routing numbers _____ _____

☐ Letter from bank official on bank letterhead indicating who has signature authority, with account and routing numbers _____ _____

New Office Supply List

FURNISHINGS AND EQUIPMENT

Waiting Room
- ☐ Chairs, 12
- ☐ End tables, 2
- ☐ Magazine racks, 2
- ☐ Books for kids and adults (discretionary)
- ☐ Pictures/art work (discretionary)
- ☐ Plants (discretionary)
- ☐ Table lamps, 2
- ☐ Patient education rack
- ☐ Wastebasket
- ☐ Computer with patient-education CD-ROM
- ☐ Computer table
- ☐ Workstation chair

Front Office
- ☐ Chairs, 4
- ☐ Printer/copier/scanner/fax machine
- ☐ Clock
- ☐ Wastebaskets, 2
- ☐ Calculators, 2
- ☐ Electric pencil sharpener
- ☐ Clipboards, 7
- ☐ Appointment book
- ☐ Petty cash box
- ☐ Locked change box
- ☐ Fire extinguisher
- ☐ Desktop computers, 2

Bathroom
- ☐ Paper towels, 1 case
- ☐ Towel dispenser
- ☐ Soap, 1 gallon
- ☐ Soap dispenser
- ☐ Toilet paper, 1 case

Employee Lounge
- ☐ Chairs, 4
- ☐ Table
- ☐ Wastebasket
- ☐ Microwave oven
- ☐ Coffee maker
- ☐ Soft drinks, 1 case
- ☐ Water cooler
- ☐ Refrigerator
- ☐ Coat rack

Physician's Office
- ☐ Desk with locking drawer
- ☐ Executive desk chair
- ☐ Side chairs, 2
- ☐ Pager
- ☐ Desk lamp
- ☐ File cabinet (four drawers)
- ☐ Dictation equipment
- ☐ Lamp
- ☐ Pictures (discretionary)
- ☐ Plants (discretionary)
- ☐ Wastebasket
- ☐ Bookcases
- ☐ Coat hook for door
- ☐ Desktop computer
- ☐ Printer

Exam/TX Rooms
- ☐ Desktop computer central to 3 exam rooms
- ☐ Exam tables, 3
- ☐ Rolling chair/stools, 3
- ☐ Side chairs, 3
- ☐ Chart holders, 3
- ☐ Cabinets, 3
- ☐ Waste receptacles (general), 3
- ☐ Waste receptacles (infectious), 3
- ☐ Coat hook and clothes hanger, 3

- ☐ Mayo stands, 3
- ☐ Otoscope, 3
- ☐ Ophthalmoscope, 3
- ☐ Gooseneck lamp, 3
- ☐ Mercury sphygmomanometer, 3
- ☐ Aneroid sphygmomanometer, 3
- ☐ Adult scale
- ☐ Pediatric scale
- ☐ Electrocardiograph
- ☐ X-ray view box, 3
- ☐ Bedpans, 6

Procedure Room
- ☐ Audiometer
- ☐ Tympanometer
- ☐ Vision screener
- ☐ Spirometer
- ☐ Holter monitor
- ☐ Flexible sigmoidoscope/supplies
- ☐ Fetal Doppler
- ☐ Adult Doppler
- ☐ Portable suction unit
- ☐ Portable O_2 unit
- ☐ Wheelchair
- ☐ Waste disposal container (general)
- ☐ Waste disposal container (infectious)
- ☐ Coat rack for door
- ☐ X-ray view box
- ☐ Exam table
- ☐ Pediatric table
- ☐ Emergency resuscitation kit
- ☐ First aid kit
- ☐ Crash cart
- ☐ Tonometer
- ☐ Ear lavage equipment
- ☐ Rolling stool
- ☐ Side chair

OFFICE SUPPLIES

- ☐ Practice management system
- ☐ 1/3-cut file folders, 3 cases
- ☐ File folder labels (plain white), 4 cases
- ☐ "Payment at time of Service" sign, 2
- ☐ Phone message pads, 2
- ☐ Post-it Notes (large and small), 2 packs
- ☐ Correction fluid, 4 containers
- ☐ Cellophane tape, 1 case (12 per case)
- ☐ Staplers, 4
- ☐ Staples, 12 boxes
- ☐ Paper clips (large and small), 12 boxes
- ☐ Copier paper, 5 reams
- ☐ Rolodex , 2
- ☐ Scissors, 2
- ☐ Glue sticks, 3

- ☐ Desk calendars, 3
- ☐ Pens (black ink), 2 dozen
- ☐ Pencils (#2), 2 dozen
- ☐ Erasers, 4
- ☐ Dictionary
- ☐ Medical dictionary
- ☐ ICD-9-CM codebook
- ☐ CPT codebook
- ☐ Vertical chart holders for desks, 2
- ☐ Scratch/note pads, 12
- ☐ Standard lined note pads, 12
- ☐ Large manila envelopes, 24
- ☐ Large rubber bands, 1 case
- ☐ Return-address stamp
- ☐ Organizers for inside desks, 3
- ☐ In and out bins, 6
- ☐ Time cards/clock (or computerized version)
- ☐ Stacking bins, 8.5 x 11-inch, for insurance desk, 10

PRINTED MATERIALS

Business
- ☐ Letterhead stationery, 2 boxes
- ☐ Letterhead envelopes, 2 boxes
- ☐ Business cards, 2 boxes
- ☐ Thank-you notes, 2 boxes
- ☐ HIPAA forms, 2 pads
- ☐ OSHA compliance package, 2 pads

- ☐ CMS 1500 forms for paper claim submission
- ☐ New patient information forms, 2 pads
- ☐ New patient medical history forms, 3 pads
- ☐ Prescription pads, 12
- ☐ Practice opening announcements, 12 pads

Medical Records
- ☐ Electronic medical record system
- ☐ Medical chart files, 5 cases
- ☐ Chart holders, 3
- ☐ Chart cabinet, 6 shelves, 3-4 ft wide
- ☐ Section dividers, 5 boxes
- ☐ Alphabetical name and year tabs, 5 boxes

CLINICAL SUPPLIES

Injections and Medications
- ☐ Medicine cups, 1000
- ☐ Insulin syringes, 2 boxes (100 per box)
- ☐ Tuberculin syringes, 2 boxes
- ☐ 1-mL syringes, 2 boxes
- ☐ 2-mL syringes, 2 boxes
- ☐ 5-mL syringes, 2 boxes
- ☐ 10-mL syringes, 2 boxes
- ☐ 27-gauge needles, 2 boxes
- ☐ 25-gauge needles, 2 boxes
- ☐ 22-gauge needles, 2 boxes
- ☐ 20-gauge needles, 2 boxes
- ☐ 18-gauge needles, 2 boxes
- ☐ Ampules or vials, 2 cases
- ☐ Sterile water, 12 500-mL bottles
- ☐ Sterile saline for injection, 6 500-mL bottles
- ☐ Sterile saline for irrigation, 6 250-mL bottles
- ☐ Alcohol wipes, 6 boxes
- ☐ Bandages, 6 boxes

- ☐ Antiseptic, 6 bottles

Instruments
- ☐ Clamps, 3
- ☐ Curettes, 3
- ☐ Forceps, 3
- ☐ Mosquitoes, 3
- ☐ Hemostats, 3
- ☐ Tissue forceps, 3
- ☐ Sutures, 1 box (12 per box)
- ☐ Needle holders, 3
- ☐ Probes, 3
- ☐ Retractors, 3
- ☐ Scalpels, 3
- ☐ Tissue scissors, 3
- ☐ Brushes for wounds, 3

Physical Examination
- ☐ Exam table paper, 5 cases
- ☐ Towels, 1 case
- ☐ Examination gowns, 5 cases

- ☐ Drapes, 5 cases
- ☐ Facial tissues, 36 boxes
- ☐ Lubricants, 3 tubes
- ☐ Flashlight, 3
- ☐ Rubber gloves, 10 boxes
- ☐ Specimen containers: urine, stool, blood, 2 cases
- ☐ Tape measure
- ☐ Tuning fork, 2
- ☐ Tongue blades, 2 boxes
- ☐ Percussion hammer

Vital Signs
- ☐ Oral thermometer, 2
- ☐ Axillary thermometer
- ☐ Rectal thermometer
- ☐ Stethoscope, 2
- ☐ Alcohol wipes, 4 boxes (200 per box)

SPECIALTY EXAM AND TREATMENTS

Eye or Ear
- ☐ Snellen eye chart
- ☐ Color plates
- ☐ Sterile eyedropper, 2
- ☐ Sterile bulb syringe, 2
- ☐ Cotton balls, 1 case
- ☐ Basins, 5
- ☐ Water thermometer

Musculoskeletal
- ☐ Bandaging, 3 boxes
- ☐ Roller bandages, 1 case
- ☐ Elastic bandages, 1 case
- ☐ Slings, 6
- ☐ Clips, 6
- ☐ Applications for heat or cold, 1 case
- ☐ Ice bag, 3
- ☐ Water bag, 2
- ☐ Washcloths, 12
- ☐ Heating pad, 2
- ☐ Protective covering, 2
- ☐ Anatomical models/charts, 1 set

Integument
- ☐ Povidone iodine, 3 16-oz bottles

- ☐ Hydrogen peroxide, 3 16-oz bottles
- ☐ Sterile 4 x 4 gauze, 1 case
- ☐ Sterile dressings, 1 box
- ☐ Sterile nonstick dressings, 1 case
- ☐ Adhesive tape, 6 rolls
- ☐ Disposable bags, 6 boxes
- ☐ Sterile ointment, 3 tubes
- ☐ Transfer forceps, 2
- ☐ Minor surgery tray, 2
- ☐ Sponges

Respiratory
- ☐ Laryngeal mirror
- ☐ Nasal dropper, 2
- ☐ Bulb syringe, 2
- ☐ Emesis basin, 6
- ☐ Nasal packing, 1 box

Cardiovascular
- ☐ Electrocardiograph paper, 2 packs
- ☐ Electrode gel, 1 tube
- ☐ ECG mounts, 2
- ☐ ECG leads and sensors, 2 boxes

Gastrointestinal
- ☐ Hemoccult tests, 1 box

- ☐ Culture and smear materials, 1 box
- ☐ Anoscope

Urinary and Male Reproductive
- ☐ Urine specimen containers, 2 cases
- ☐ Urinometer
- ☐ Reagent strips, 1 bottle
- ☐ Midstream urine containers, 2 cases
- ☐ Slides, 2 boxes
- ☐ Culture medium plates, 2
- ☐ Sterile applicators, 1 box
- ☐ Sterile swabs, 1 box
- ☐ Fixative
- ☐ Clean catch instructions

Female Reproductive
- ☐ Vaginal speculum, 2 boxes
- ☐ Applicator, 1 box
- ☐ Slides, 2 boxes
- ☐ Pap fixative KOH solution
- ☐ Perineal pads, 1 box
- ☐ Uterine dressing forceps
- ☐ Fetoscope
- ☐ Diaphragm fitting rings

PLEASE READ

NOTICE TO PATIENTS OF [INSERT PRACTICE NAME]

Under [insert state] law, physicians are generally required to carry medical malpractice insurance or otherwise demonstrate financial responsibility to cover potential claims for medical malpractice.

The physicians employed by [practice name] have decided not to carry
medical malpractice insurance.
This is permitted under [insert state] law subject to certain conditions. [Insert state] law imposes
strict penalties against noninsured physicians who fail to satisfy adverse judgments arising from
claims of medical malpractice. This notice is provided pursuant to [insert state] law. Should you
have any questions regarding this matter, please contact [responsible person].

Overall Practice Self-Assessment Tool

Check if Completed		Responsible Party	Notes

Assess the Physical Layout's Condition

☐ Cleanliness and appearance _____ _____

☐ Practice layout _____ _____

☐ Location _____ _____

☐ Reception and intake _____ _____

☐ Exam room and patient flow patterns _____ _____

☐ Billing and administrative area _____ _____

☐ Fire and safety plans _____ _____

☐ Notice of privacy _____ _____

☐ Mission statement _____ _____

☐ Descriptive data about the facility _____ _____

   ☐ Brochures _____ _____

   ☐ Pamphlets _____ _____

   ☐ Media articles related to the physician practice _____ _____

   ☐ Press releases or newspaper announcements _____ _____

   ☐ Other marketing materials used to promote the practice _____ _____

Personnel Records

☐ HR policies and procedures _____ _____

☐ Resume and applications _____ _____

☐ Review personnel file documentation _____ _____

☐ Licenses _____ _____

☐ I-9 forms _____ _____

☐ Social Security records _____ _____

Check if Completed		Responsible Party	Notes

Personnel (continued)

☐	Application for employment	_____	_____
☐	Tax withholding forms	_____	_____
☐	Employee evaluation forms	_____	_____
☐	Hepatitis waivers	_____	_____
☐	OSHA standards training records	_____	_____
☐	State biomedical waste plan training records	_____	_____
☐	HIPAA privacy forms	_____	_____
☐	http://www.epls.gov/epls/search.do	_____	_____
☐	OIG Web list (http://exclusions.oig.hhs.gov)	_____	_____
☐	Pension and benefits forms	_____	_____

Billing and Administrative Areas

☐	Health information management policy	_____	_____
☐	Record maintenance and security protocols	_____	_____
☐	Billing management software contracts	_____	_____
☐	Recall system	_____	_____
☐	Physician query system	_____	_____
☐	Billing training materials	_____	_____
☐	Patient records management	_____	_____

Historical Financial Data

| ☐ | Historical financial data, including income statements, balance sheets, cash flow statements and notes, if applicable, for the past 3 years | _____ | _____ |
| ☐ | Revenue detail listing by payer for capitated revenue, fee-for-service, stop loss, shared risk, and other income in an absolute dollar amount and as a percentage of total revenue for the past 3 years | _____ | _____ |

Check if Completed		Responsible Party	Notes

Historical Financial Data (continued)

☐ Internally prepared reports that include statements by payer, member months, capitation rates by payer, gross charges, net collections and adjustments, and payer mixes for the past 3 years   _____   _____

☐ Internally prepared statistics related to practice operations and performance for the past 3 years (often available through a computer software program)   _____   _____

☐ Annual and usage statistics for the past year and year to date, encompassing that by payer and physician, including summary totals   _____   _____

☐ Summary of fee-for-service revenue and data concerning number of patient visits for the last 3 years per service-service patient   _____   _____

☐ Summary of physicians' by specialty at the practice, including their guaranteed compensation, total production, and net collections for the past 3 years   _____   _____

☐ Summary of medical services provided by the practice (eg, ancillary services, radiology, laboratory).   _____   _____

☐ Review of the balance sheet and summary of any "hidden assets"   _____   _____

☐ Summary of rental costs for the practice. If the practice owns the facility, obtain or perform an analysis of the effective cost per square foot for occupancy.   _____   _____

☐ Summary of bad debt write-offs and patient refunds for the past 2 years and current year-to-date   _____   _____

☐ Accounts receivable management reports for the current and previous year, as follows:
    a. Accounts receivable summary
    b. Aging reports by payer
    c. Aged credit balance   _____   _____

Check if Completed		Responsible Party	Notes

Contracts and Agreements

☐ Copies of physicians' employment agreements and contracts. If the practice is a partnership, limited liability corporation, or limited liability partnership, obtain agreements or articles of incorporation.   _____   _____

☐ Copies of all third-party payer and management service contracts and licenses   _____   _____

☐ List of all current agreements, as follows: _____   _____

     ☐ Equipment leases   _____   _____

     ☐ Real estate leases   _____   _____

     ☐ Licenses   _____   _____

     ☐ Contracts from supply vendors   _____   _____

     ☐ Service and maintenance contracts on equipment   _____   _____

     ☐ All other applicable contracts   _____   _____

☐ General, corporate, or physician entity data   _____   _____

☐ Number of active patients for each of the last 3 years   _____   _____

☐ Number of new patients in each of the last 3 years (preferably, separated by payer, eg, fee-for-service vs capitated)   _____   _____

☐ Analyze and obtain physician compensation and bonus arrangements, including perquisites   _____   _____

☐ Average number of hours worked per week for each physician for current and previous 3 years and practice hours noting before 8:00 AM and after 5:00 PM availability   _____   _____

☐ Average number of office visits per month for each physician for current year and previous 3 years   _____   _____

Check if Completed		Responsible Party	Notes

Contracts and Agreements (continued)

☐ Current schedules of each physician, detailing the physician's practice sites and hours available each day of the week for appointment scheduling   _____   _____

☐ Details of buy-sell agreements within the physician partners   _____   _____

☐ Details of benefits, including retirement plans, stock options, bonus, and profit sharing plans within the practice, covering physicians and the current employees   _____   _____

☐ Organization charts showing each physician's title and employees' responsibilities, including any crossover of employee functions   _____   _____

☐ Further summary of practice personnel, including the following: _____   _____

    ☐ Number of full-time employees (FTEs) by department or specialty   _____   _____

    ☐ Average salary for each department denoting full-time vs part-time employees and an average cost per year for each position   _____   _____

    ☐ Payroll details by individual (rate per hour or salary for the current year; overtime worked and paid)   _____   _____

☐ Details of any outstanding liabilities to or from the officers, directors, and stockholders of the corporation or partners depending on the structure of the legal entity.   _____   _____

☐ Summary of outstanding debt, including lending institution, maturity terms, current interest rate, and loan covenants; a breakdown of short-term vs long-term debt; discussion of past, current, or anticipated litigation or contingent liabilities, including all potential environmental liabilities. Major emphasis of this analysis applies to historical and current malpractice claims.   _____   _____

Check if Completed		Responsible Party	Notes

Contracts and Agreements (continued)

☐ Copies of all significant reports compiled by third parties and to what extent they accepted and carried out the plans, including:

    ☐ Marketing studies

    ☐ Strategic plans

    ☐ Other appraisal reports (eg, tangible assets only, intangibles, business enterprises, or real estate)

☐ Summary of computer systems, entailing hardware, software, capacity, functions, and the extent of services provided within the system (eg, billing, accounting, payroll, patient scheduling)

☐ Utilization review policy and referral authorizations for the physicians

☐ List of nearby hospitals and those where the physicians have active staff privileges

☐ Summary of hospital activity within the practice, including inpatient and outpatient admissions and any other direct relationships (such as medical directorships)

☐ Summary of closest competitors (usually, practices within a designated radius, depending on population density)

☐ Summary of the physical layout of the offices, preferably including a copy of the actual floor plan blueprint or, at least, a detailed drawing or diagram

☐ Summary of the practice's rooms, including waiting area, examining rooms, offices, procedure rooms, restrooms, storage rooms, laboratory areas, radiology, etc

☐ Summary of outstanding claims relating to employees, such as workers' compensation or EEOC claims pending, and a list of all claims settled over the past 3 years

Check if Completed		Responsible Party	Notes

Contracts and Agreements (continued)

☐   Summary of all insurance coverage pertaining to the practice (eg, professional and general liability, and property and casualty insurance)   _____   _____

Stockholder/Owner Information for a Corporation

☐   Copies of all corporate stock certificates   _____   _____

☐   Buy-sell option or repurchase agreements   _____   _____

☐   Options authorized or granted   _____   _____

☐   List of all shareholders, copies of stock certificates, including number of shares held by each stockholder, and percentage equity interest of each shareholder.   _____   _____

☐   Summary of historical stock transactions   _____   _____

☐   A schedule of dividends accrued and paid   _____   _____

Stockholder/Owner Information for a Partnership or Similar Entity (eg, Limited Liability Company)

☐   Copies of the partnership agreement   _____   _____

☐   Summary of partnership agreement activity, additions, deletions   _____   _____

☐   Summary of distributions, bonuses, changes in partners' compensation   _____   _____

☐   JCAHO Readiness and Survey Reports   _____   _____

☐   HIPAA and other training materials and reports   _____   _____

☐   Biohazardous waste policies and training records   _____   _____

☐   DRG audits and training materials   _____   _____

☐   Security and privacy practices   _____   _____

Practice Promotion and Marketing

Check if Completed	Promotional or Marketing Strategy	Responsible Party	Notes
☐	Reserve office phone number, if possible, or determine answering service phone number.	_____	_____
☐	Find out the date when phone books are printed.	_____	_____
☐	Have your name listed in the telephone book, white and yellow pages.	_____	_____
☐	Notify area pharmacies that you are starting a practice.	_____	_____
☐	Place newspaper ads about opening.	_____	_____
☐	Arrange to give talks to community groups on health topics.	_____	_____
☐	Notify drug detail people and appropriate salespeople that you are setting up practice.	_____	_____
☐	Talk with social service and other referring agencies (eg, home health care agencies) about the services to be provided.	_____	_____
☐	Check if there is a patient referral service available through the local medical society or hospital and provide them with essential information.	_____	_____
☐	Consider memberships in civic and church organizations.	_____	_____

Expense	January	February	March	April	May	June	July	August	September	October	November	December	Total
Accounting													
Advertising													
Auto expenses													
Bank charges													
Build out—contractor													
Engineer													
Collection expenses													
Computer													
Contract aer admin													
Continuing ed													
Dues and licenses													
Equip lease													
Furniture—office													
Furniture—medical													
Insurance—health													
Bad debts													
Insurance—malprac													
Insurance—office													
Insurance—work comp													
Lab													
Legal & acct													
Loan for start-up													
PCs													
Practice mgmt cons													
Depletion													
Licenses													
Meals													
Misc expenses													
Outside services													
Postage													
Rent													
Repairs & maint													
Salaries													
Subscriptions													
Supplies—medical													
Supplies—office													
Taxes—payroll													
Taxes—property													
Travel													
Telephone													
Utilities													
Total Expenses													

Created: [Date]

Professional Insurance Needs Checklist

Check if Completed		Responsible Party	Notes
☐	Business owner's policy	_____	_____
☐	Office overhead	_____	_____
☐	Business interruption	_____	_____
☐	Nonowned automobile	_____	_____
☐	Premises liability	_____	_____
☐	Equipment floater	_____	_____
☐	Malpractice	_____	_____
☐	Employer's liability	_____	_____
☐	Employee fidelity bond	_____	_____
☐	Office contents	_____	_____
☐	Umbrella: Provides comprehensive catastrophic liability coverage for liability claims beyond the limits of regular disability programs.	_____	_____
☐	Workers' compensation: Required by law and is determined on a state-by-state basis. Check with your state's Workers' Compensation Board Industrial Commission.	_____	_____
☐	Health: Major medical for yourself and employees	_____	_____
☐	Disability	_____	_____
☐	Life	_____	_____
☐	Automobile	_____	_____

Reference Books and Materials

Check if Completed	Books and Materials	Responsible Party	Notes
☐	*Medical Practice Policies & Procedures* www.amabookstore.com	_____	_____
☐	HIPAA compliance plan	_____	_____
☐	Obtain/develop written bloodborne pathogens and TB exposure control plan in compliance with OSHA (www.osha.gov)	_____	_____
☐	Procedure coding book(s) (CPT codebooks)	_____	_____
☐	Diagnostic coding book(s)	_____	_____
☐	Insurance claim forms	_____	_____
☐	Current Medicare handbook and fee schedule	_____	_____
☐	Preliminary job descriptions for employees	_____	_____
☐	Policy manual for your employees	_____	_____

Selecting and Equipping a New Practice

Check if Completed		Number Needed	Notes
☐	Perform a market analysis of where to open practice.	_____	_____
☐	Visit banks and "shop" for a loan, if needed.	_____	_____
☐	Check sites for leasing/buying medical office space.	_____	_____
☐	Check zoning ordinances with your local city hall and/or zoning board regarding signage, type of businesses allowed in the area, and ask about any anticipated changes.	_____	_____
☐	Check on utility requirements for the office.	_____	_____
☐	Coordinate with developer and hospital.	_____	_____
☐	If leasing, see if any leasehold improvements are needed and when you can start making these improvements.	_____	_____
☐	Determine office layout and design.	_____	_____
☐	Determine office and medical equipment needed. If installing x-ray equipment, check with the regulatory agencies. Same checks should be made for laboratory and outpatient surgery facilities.	_____	_____
☐	Determine likely office hours on the basis of community needs.	_____	_____

Electronic Systems to Operate Practice

☐	Dictating machine	_____	_____
☐	Intercom system	_____	_____
☐	Photocopy machine	_____	_____
☐	PCs	_____	_____
☐	Network	_____	_____
☐	Fax machine	_____	_____
☐	Telephone system	_____	_____

Check if
Completed   Number Needed   Notes

Electronic Systems to Operate Practice (continued)

☐   Adding machine   _____   _____

☐   Light signaling system   _____   _____

Reception Area Furniture

☐   Chairs   _____   _____

☐   Tables   _____   _____

☐   Lamps   _____   _____

☐   Magazine racks   _____   _____

☐   Decide on and order magazines for   _____   _____
     reception room.

☐   Decide on and order medical journals   _____   _____
     for yourself.

Business Office Furniture

☐   Secretarial chairs for employees   _____   _____

☐   Chairs for patients for any type of   _____   _____
     consultation

☐   Desks, unless built-in counter space   _____   _____
     is available

☐   Standard pull-out files for assorted   _____   _____
     business records

☐   Files for office charts   _____   _____

☐   Tape calculators (machines that can   _____   _____
     multiply, divide, and store information,
     as well as add and subtract and print it
     on paper for bookkeepers)

☐   Waste receptacle   _____   _____

☐   Telephone   _____   _____

☐   Tables on which to place computer and   _____   _____
     printer if these are to be used

☐   Photocopier   _____   _____

☐   Postage machine   _____   _____

Check if Completed		Number Needed	Notes

Business Office Furniture (continued)

☐ Storage cabinet for supplies

☐ Transcription equipment

☐ Wall decorations

Consultation Room

☐ Desk and executive chair

☐ Visitor chairs

☐ Cabinct for private files

☐ Bookshelves

☐ Dictating equipment

☐ Telephone

☐ Calculator

☐ Wall decorations

Examination Room

☐ Examination table

☐ Desk chair

☐ Doctor's stool

☐ Hangers and clothing hooks

☐ Mirror and supply cabinet

☐ Wall decorations

☐ Otoscope

☐ Sphygmomanometer

☐ Ophthalmoscope

☐ Other medical instruments

Check if Completed		Number Needed	Notes

Laboratory

☐ Refrigerator

☐ Stools on which patients and /or technician may sit while blood is drawn

☐ Various supply cabinets

☐ Small-size file for laboratory/business records

☐ Telephone

☐ Necessary laboratory instruments

X-ray Room

☐ X-ray table

☐ X-ray processor/developer

Nurses' Station

☐ Counter space (built in or added)

☐ Telephone

☐ Pigeon-hole cupboard for charts, charge and laboratory slips

☐ Rooms for storage and/or adequate shelving

Kitchen/Break Room

☐ Table and chairs

☐ Refrigerator

☐ Microwave oven

☐ Coffee maker

☐ Telephone

EMR Assessment Questionnaire and Request for Proposal Vendor Questionnaire

Clinic Name

Vendor:
Date:
Contact:
Contact telephone:
Contact e-mail:

EMR Assessment Questionnaire

Answer each of the following questions regarding your EMR needs by checking Yes or No.

Chart Organization

Yes ☐ No ☐   1.   Do you want a patient's electronic chart to contain all patient data, or do paper items still need to be kept in the office?

Yes ☐ No ☐   2.   Do you want all patient information available in one area (ie, a physician only needs to look up the files once)?

Yes ☐ No ☐   3.   Do you want the EMR to offer a "single screen" summary of the problem lists, allergies, medications, and prevention prompts?

Yes ☐ No ☐   4.   Do you want the record to be accessed during patient visits?

Yes ☐ No ☐   5.   Please indicate whether you want the EMR chart to contain the following sections or features:

Yes ☐ No ☐   a.   Chart summary

Yes ☐ No ☐   b.   Past medical history

Yes ☐ No ☐   c.   Past social history

Yes ☐ No ☐   d.   Family history

Yes ☐ No ☐   e.   Progress notes

Yes ☐ No ☐   f.   Images (radiological, sonographic, ultrasonic)

Yes ☐ No ☐   g.   Current medications

Yes ☐ No ☐   h.   Ineffective medication list

Yes ☐ No ☐   i.   Historical medication list

Yes ☐ No ☐   j.   Formulary checking

Yes ☐ No ☐   k.   Drug interaction checking

Yes ☐ No ☐   l.   Allergy interaction checking

Yes ☐ No ☐   m.   Problem list

Yes ☐ No ☐   n.   Lab results

Yes ☐ No ☐   o.   Problem lists

Yes ☐ No ☐   p.   Messages associated with the patient

Yes ☐ No ☐   q.   Health maintenance (this section should alert physicians when a patient is overdue for certain procedures)

Yes ☐ No ☐   r.   Letters associated with the patient

Yes ☐ No ☐   s.   Disease- and problem-specific flow charts

Yes ☐ No ☐   t.   Customizable chart sections that can hold other textual data that do not fit in any of the premade chart sections.

Yes ☐ No ☐   6.   Do you want the chart to contain alerts that appear every time the chart is opened?

Yes ☐ No ☐   7.   Do you want the medication section to contain different flags that appear every time the medication section is opened?

Yes ☐ No ☐   8.   Do you want all numerical data in the chart to be graphed?

Yes ☐ No ☐   9.   Do you want the user to be able to create flow sheets with data fields populated from other data in the record (NOT requiring redundant entry)?

Yes ☐ No ☐   10.   Do you want physicians to be able to electronically review and sign progress notes with forwarding capability for electronic review and cosignatures?

Yes ☐ No ☐   11.   Do you want the chart to be viewed from a remote location (ie, the physician's home or the hospital)?

Yes ☐ No ☐   12.   Do you want medication lists automatically updated as medications are prescribed?

Yes ☐ No ☐   13.   Do you want drug instructions to be printed for a patient?

Yes ☐ No ☐   14.   Do you want prescriptions to be faxed to the pharmacy or printed at the physician's discretion?

Yes ☐ No ☐   15.   Do you want the EMR to create growth charts?

Documentation

Yes ☐ No ☐   16.   Do you want the EMR to support free text–based input?

Yes ☐ No ☐   17.   Do you want it to support pick list–based input?

Yes ☐ No ☐   18.   Do you want it to support the use of progress note templates?

Yes ☐ No ☐   19.   Do you want it to support insertion of previous progress notes into a new note?

Yes ☐ No ☐   20.   Do you want it to support the input of predefined pieces of text (similar to macros in Microsoft Word)?

Yes ☐ No ☐   21.   Do you want it to support the use of voice recognition software to record a note?

Yes ☐ No ☐   22.   Do you want the EMR to build "required fields" into a note to force better documentation?

Yes ☐ No ☐   23.   Do you want the EMR to have a built-in spell checker?

Yes ☐ No ☐   24.   Do you want all information entered into progress notes to be automatically used to update the entire chart so that no dual entry is required?

Yes ☐ No ☐   25.   Do you want it to support the uploading of transcribed notes directly into the chart?

Yes ☐ No ☐   26.   Do you want uploaded transcribed notes to update ALL sections of the chart?

Yes ☐ No ☐   27.   Do you want vitals signs, allergies, current medications, and past medical and social histories, etc, to be imported into current progress note?

Yes ☐ No ☐   28.   Do you want progress notes to have hyperlinks built in to retrieve external files?

Yes ☐ No ☐   29.   Do you want physicians to be able to document multiple problems within the same progress note?

Yes ☐ No ☐   30.   Do you want progress notes to support multiple signatures for midlevels?

Yes ☐ No ☐   31.   Do you want progress notes to be sorted by clinic, physician, or specialty?

Yes ☐ No ☐   32.   Do you want images to be attached to a progress note?

Yes ☐ No ☐   33.   Do you want physicians to be able to add free text anywhere within the note?

Yes ☐ No ☐   34.   Do you want the signing of a note to require an electronic signature that is separate and different from the application password?

Yes ☐ No ☐   35.   Do you want the problem list to be hyperlinked to related progress notes?

Yes ☐ No ☐   36.   Do you want the EMR to include prebuilt progress note templates? If so, how many?

Yes ☐ No ☐   37.   Do you want users to be able to modify existing templates and create new templates without programming skills?

Yes ☐ No ☐   38.   Do you want the EMR to contain patient education materials?

Yes ☐ No ☐   39.   If so, do you want users to be able to attach patient education materials to relevant progress note templates?

Yes ☐ No ☐   40.   Do you want the progress note templates to be linked to the appropriate ICD-9-CM or ICD-10-CM and CPT codes?

Workflow Tools

Yes ☐ No ☐   41.   Do you want the EMR to contain a clinic-wide e-mail/messaging system?

Yes ☐ No ☐   42.   Do you want the charts to be attached to the messages?

Yes ☐ No ☐   43.   Do you want the messages to be recorded in the chart for documentation?

Yes ☐ No ☐   44.   Do you want urgent messages to be highlighted in a different color?

Yes ☐ No ☐   45.   Do you want a user's messages to be available from any workstation to which they are logged on?

Yes ☐ No ☐   46.   Do you want the system to contain a letter-writing tool?

Yes ☐ No ☐   47.   Do you want users to create templates for letters that automatically bring patient data into the letters (eg, lab values or current medications)?

Yes ☐ No ☐   48. Do you want the system to have an electronic in-box that physicians can open to review unsigned notes or lab results?

Yes ☐ No ☐   49. Upon signing results or notes, do you want the documents to be forwarded to other physicians in the clinic?

Yes ☐ No ☐   50. Do you want the EMR to create chart summary reports?

Yes ☐ No ☐   a.   By individual patient

Yes ☐ No ☐   b.   For scheduled patients

Yes ☐ No ☐   c.   Patients seen on a particular day

Yes ☐ No ☐   d.   All patients for to a primary physician

Yes ☐ No ☐   e.   Patients on a list generated by patient inquiry

Yes ☐ No ☐   f.   All patients within the system

Yes ☐ No ☐   51. Do you want the EMR to have built-in reports to find the following?

Yes ☐ No ☐   a.   Unsigned progress notes

Yes ☐ No ☐   b.   Unsaved progress notes

Yes ☐ No ☐   c.   Missing progress notes

Yes ☐ No ☐   52. Do you want the EMR to have a search feature that can search for a combination of criteria?

Yes ☐ No ☐   53. If so, up to how many different data elements can the search feature use to select data?

Yes ☐ No ☐   54. Do you want data retrieved by the search feature to be exported?

Yes ☐ No ☐   55. Do you want all data to be exported?

Security

Yes ☐ No ☐   56. Do you want different users to have different levels of security?

Yes ☐ No ☐   57. Do you want certain users to have view-only access to parts of the chart?

Yes ☐ No ☐   58. How many security settings do you want the application to have?

Yes ☐ No ☐   59. Do you want them to be able to be modified by persons with the appropriate security level?

Yes ☐ No ☐   60. Do you want certain users to be denied access to certain chart sections but not the rest of the chart in order to maintain confidentiality?

Integration and Interfacing

Yes ☐ No ☐   61. Do you want a scheduling program that can be integrated with the EMR?

Yes ☐ No ☐   62. If so, what features result in this integration?

Yes ☐ No ☐   63. Do you want a billing program that can be integrated with the EMR?

Yes ☐ No ☐   64. If so, what features result in this integration?

Yes ☐ No ☐   65. Do you want the EMR to interface with laboratories so that lab results are brought directly into the system?

Yes ☐ No ☐   66. If so, which labs can be included in the interface?

Yes ☐ No ☐   67. Do you want the EMR to interface to other practice management products if so desired?

Yes ☐ No ☐   68. Do you want any other products or tools (eg, MS Office) integrated into your EMR?

Support

Yes ☐ No ☐   69. What hours of availability for technical support do you need?

Yes ☐ No ☐   70. How many employees dedicated to support do you need?

Yes ☐ No ☐   71. How do customers access technical support? Email? Telephone? On site?

Yes ☐ No ☐   72. What are the recommended backup procedures and their frequencies?

Yes ☐ No ☐   73. What kind of problem escalation procedures do you need?

Vendor Questionnaire
Corporate Information

I. **Company History**
  A. Give a brief overview of the history of your company.
  B. How long has your company been in business?
  C. Provide brief biographies of the officers/principals of your company.
  D. Highlight the involvement of physicians or other clinicians in the development of your products.
  E. Provide a statement attesting to the stability of your company.
  F. Does your company have a parent organization? If so, please provide a brief description of that organization.
  G. Is the EMR application your company's main product? If not, please describe the main product(s).
  H. Please describe your company's mission.
  I. Please describe your company's experience with implementing EMRs.
  J. What distinguishes your company from your competitors?
  K. Please list all organizations and companies that have formed a partnership agreement with your company. Include a brief description of each one.

II. **Company Organization**
  A. Company geography
    1. Address of corporate headquarters
    2. Number of national locations
  B. Employees
    1. Number of total employees
    2. Number of employees dedicated to support
    3. Number of employees dedicated to implementation and training
    4. Number of employees dedicated to development
  C. Company contact information
    1. Web site
    2. Corporate phone number
    3. Corporate fax number

III. **Finances**
  A. Is your company publicly or privately held?
  B. How long has your company been profitable?
  C. What was your revenue for last year?

IV. **Usage**
  A. How many practices currently use your products?
  B. How many users currently use your products?
  C. What types of organizations use your products?
  D. How many sites did you install within the past year?
  E. Please provide three references of similar size and specialty including the following information on each
    1. Name of the practice
    2. Address
    3. Number of physicians using your EMR
    4. Specialty
    5. Number of sites
    6. Contact name and position
    7. Telephone or e-mail address

V. **Product Information: Technical Requirements**
  A. What type of server is recommended?
  B. What operating system is recommended for the server?
  C. What type of workstation is recommended?

    D.   What operating system is recommended for the workstations?
    E.   What databases can be used with your EMR?
    F.   Do you have users running the application on a wireless network?

VI. **Product Information: General (address each of the following with regard to your EMR)**
    A.   Reliability
    B.   Scalability
    C.   Cost-effectiveness
    D.   Ease of use

VII. **Reporting**
    A.   Can the EMR create chart summary reports?
        1.   By individual patient
        2.   For scheduled patients
        3.   Patients seen on a particular day
        4.   All patients for a primary physician
        5.   Patients on a list generated by patient inquiry
        6.   All patients within the system
    B.   Does the EMR have built-in reports to find the following:
        1.   Unsigned progress notes
        2.   Unsaved progress notes
        3.   Missing progress notes
    C.   Does the EMR have a search feature that can search for a combination of criteria?
    D.   If so, up to how many different data elements can the search feature use to select data?
    E.   Can data retrieved by the search feature be exported?
    F.   Can all data be exported?

VIII. **Implementation**
    A.   Please describe your implementation process.

IX. **Pricing**
    A.   Please include a price quote for the proposed system.

New Practice Start-up

Check if Completed		Responsible Party	Notes
☐	If not licensed, contact state medical licensing board.	_____	_____

☐	Assemble team of advisors (as appropriate):
	  Attorney
	  Banker
	  Accountant
	  Management consultant
	  Insurance broker
	  Real estate broker
	  Physician mentor
		_____	_____

☐	Prepare income/expenditure projection for first year of practice.	_____	_____
☐	Apply for your federal employer ID number (fill out form #SS-4).	_____	_____
☐	Acquire checking account—personal.	_____	_____
☐	Acquire checking account—business.	_____	_____
☐	Acquire savings accounts—personal and business.	_____	_____
☐	Consider a money market fund—open directly or through a stockbroker.	_____	_____
☐	Arrange for accepting credit cards.	_____	_____
☐	Obtain CLIA registration AHCA. Must have CLIA number to bill lab work of moderate complexity or above or a waived certificate if not performing testing above the waived level. Keep photocopy of your application as proof you have applied.	_____	_____
☐	Determine whether your state also requires separate licensure.	_____	_____
☐	Obtain county and city occupational business license.	_____	_____
☐	Evaluate office lease and/or partnership agreement contracts with your attorney before you sign them.	_____	_____
☐	Decide on Medicare participant status and send in paperwork with provider application.	_____	_____
☐	Hire key office employee.	_____	_____

Check if Completed		Responsible Party	Notes
☐	Organization form—sole proprietor or corporation?	_____	_____
☐	Stationery and logo (corporate identity on everything)	_____	_____
☐	Signage (corporate name, logo, etc)	_____	_____
☐	Develop practice goals and plans.	_____	_____
☐	Inter-physician agreements	_____	_____
☐	Obtain bids on major office equipment. Compare lease vs purchase. Be sure to get guarantee of delivery date and in-transit insurance.	_____	_____
☐	Select computer billing system.	_____	_____
☐	Select electronic medical records system.	_____	_____
☐	Obtain the services of an answering service: Physician's exchange (hospital) Personal (office) Cell phones	_____	_____
☐	Order medical records systems, if not electronic.	_____	_____
☐	Accounts payable bookkeeping	_____	_____
☐	Accounting bookkeeping system	_____	_____
☐	Payroll issues	_____	_____
☐	Order sign for the office.	_____	_____
☐	Obtain office supplies.	_____	_____
☐	Arrange for telephone installation.	_____	_____
☐	Write your state department of labor for state employment regulations and wage and hour information.	_____	_____
☐	Check local resources for personnel (eg, newspapers, training schools, employment web sites)	_____	_____
☐	Apply for your state employer identification number.	_____	_____

Check if Completed		Responsible Party	Notes
☐	Review accounting and tax procedures with consultant (payroll procedures, deposits balanced to income, division of money handling duties, etc).	_____	_____
☐	Obtain "Small Business Tax Guide" and your federal estimated income tax form through your state employment office or labor department or through an accountant.	_____	_____
☐	Obtain payroll withholding booklets (federal, state, city) through your local IRS office or accountant's office.	_____	_____
☐	Plan and order appointment scheduling book, if not using computerized scheduling.	_____	_____
☐	Arrange for, as needed: Janitorial services Laundry services Grass Mowing	_____	_____
☐	Order clinical supplies.	_____	_____
☐	Order business supplies: Appointment cards Business cards Patient recall systems Letterhead, stationery, and envelopes Stationery supplies Deposit stamp for checks Prescription pads	_____	_____
☐	Interview/meet with the local collection agencies.	_____	_____
☐	Decide on collection/Insurance policy.	_____	_____
☐	Obtain preprinted telephone message pads.	_____	_____
☐	ON OPENING—Have utilities turned on: Electricity Gas Water	_____	_____
☐	Get patient information printed.	_____	_____
☐	Hang out shingle.	_____	_____
☐	Establish a petty cash fund.	_____	_____
☐	Establish a change fund.	_____	_____

Check if Completed		Responsible Party	Notes

Accounting Items to Review as Practice Opens

☐   Payroll procedures
        a. Annotations
        b. Advances
        c. 941 deposits
_____   _____

☐   Check writing from office account
        —descriptions
_____   _____

☐   Bank deposits—balance to income.
        Receipts deposited in full with each deposit.
_____   _____

☐   Practice activity & cash journal—and daily
        routine. Be sure to list deposits individually
        on journal and in check stub. Do not combine
        multiple deposits into one amount in check
        register on journal.
_____   _____

☐   W-4s to each new employee—first day
        of work
_____   _____

☐   Form I-9
_____   _____

☐   Change fund—$300 in small bills.
        Separate from petty cash fund. Swap big
        bills from cash on hand for small bills as
        needed. Change fund will be $300 at end of
        each day. Take big bills to bank and exchange
        for small bills as needed.
        Replenish writing check to petty cash.
_____   _____

☐   Professional gift giving limits—currently
        $25 per person, per year
_____   _____

☐   Professional entertainment—recordkeeping
        rules (who, what, where, why, when)
_____   _____

☐   Travel expenses and recordkeeping
        a. Auto log & standard mileage rate = 50.5 cents per mile for 2008
        b. What's deductible when you take a trip/vacation?
        c. Accountable plan
        d. Documentation
_____   _____

Check if Completed		Responsible Party	Notes
	Items to Review as Practice Open		
☐	8109 tax payment coupons	_____	_____
☐	Circular E	_____	_____
☐	Cash journal	_____	_____
☐	W-4s	_____	_____

Board of Directors Listing

[CLIENT NAME]

There are [enter number] members of the Board of Directors of [Client Name] _____ d/b/a
_____(   ).

[Client] owns the [Client Name]. The directors are as follows:

_____

_____   _____

Home   **Home**

Other Administrative Officers for [Client Name]

_____   _____

Administrative Director   Clinical Director

Organizational Chart

[CLIENT NAME]

BOARD OF DIRECTORS

[DEPARTMENT]   [DEPARTMENT]   [DEPARTMENT]   [DEPARTMENT]

chapter 2

Practice Organization

In addition to the practice of medicine, physicians also need knowledge and skill in the business of medicine. Issues related to incorporation, finances, human resources, purchasing decisions, and local, state, and federal laws, rules, regulations, and ordinances affect everyday practice and the short- and long-term success of the business. This chapter provides forms, checklists, and templates to assist in the organization of a practice.

Selecting and evaluating personnel, including associate physicians, physician assistants, and nurse practitioners, are some of the most important tasks in practice organization. This chapter includes an evaluation form for a midlevel practitioner that can also be used in employee selection. In addition, the form could be adapted to other positions in the practice.

In today's health care marketplace, the need to be accredited as a medical practice is becoming more common. Some insurance carriers are eliminating their own credentialing departments and looking to established accrediting bodies, such as the AAAHC, AAHC, and JCHAO, with standardized criteria to provide such services. To be accredited, the medical practice needs to demonstrate compliance with developed standards of care *and* standards of business practice. The template for a corporate information outline in this chapter is designed to help practices organize the required information.

Other tools provided in this chapter to assist with organization of a practice are a template for an organizational chart and a form for board of director listings for practices that include more than one professional.

When the time comes to close or relocate a practice, various agencies and individuals need to be notified. A checklist for closing a practice and a sample letter to patients are included in the chapter.

Tools for Practice Organization

Number	Title	Purpose	Notes
02001	Form for an Associate Physician, Physician Assistant, or Nurse Practitioner Evaluation	To evaluate a provider's performance	This tool can be used when selecting a new midlevel or evaluating a current provider.
02002	Checklist for Closing a Practice	Closing a practice requires as much attention to detail as does opening a practice. The checklist assists in managing that process.	This checklist identifies not only the steps involved in closing a practice because of retirement, but also the agencies and individuals who should be notified.
02003	Template for a Discontinuation of Practice Letter	To notify patients of practice closure	This letter can be used to inform patients of discontinuation of a medical practice; it also permits patients to designate a new physician and consent to your provision of records to the new physician. The letter could be adapted to inform the medical community of retirement or relocation.

Associate Physician, Physician Assistant, or Nurse Practitioner Evaluation

Employee Name: _____

Evaluation Performed By: _____ Date: _____

Evaluation Received By: _____ Date: _____

Period: from _____ to _____ Next Review Due: _____

	Excellent	Very Good	Good	Average	Poor	N/A	Comments
Interpersonal Skills							
With lay staff	1	2	3	4	5	6	
With referring physicians	1	2	3	4	5	6	
With hospital medical staff	1	2	3	4	5	6	
With professional, technical, and lay staff	1	2	3	4	5	6	
Clinical Performance							
Demonstrates knowledge/skill	1	2	3	4	5	6	
Demonstrates diagnostic ability	1	2	3	4	5	6	
Proper chart documentation	1	2	3	4	5	6	
Patient privacy compliance	1	2	3	4	5	6	
Continuing education	1	2	3	4	5	6	
Practice Development							
Generates new patients	1	2	3	4	5	6	
Retains existing patients	1	2	3	4	5	6	
Develops referral relationships	1	2	3	4	5	6	
Practice marketing	1	2	3	4	5	6	
Suggests practice improvements	1	2	3	4	5	6	
Day-to-Day Practice							
Relationship with patients	1	2	3	4	5	6	
On time to office	1	2	3	4	5	6	

	Excellent	Very Good	Good	Average	Poor	N/A	Comments
Charts/referring letters/dictation	1	2	3	4	5	6	
Billing information	1	2	3	4	5	6	
Telephone effectiveness	1	2	3	4	5	6	
Practice Style							
Work ethic/production	1	2	3	4	5	6	
Utilization/cost-effectiveness/efficiency	1	2	3	4	5	6	
Enthusiasm	1	2	3	4	5	6	
Flexibility	1	2	3	4	5	6	
Performance under pressure	1	2	3	4	5	6	
Miscellaneous							
Assistance in practice management	1	2	3	4	5	6	
Support of practice goals	1	2	3	4	5	6	

Signature of Employee: _____ **Date:** _____

Signature of Reviewer: _____ **Date:** _____

Closing a Practice at Retirement

Check if Completed		Responsible Party	Notes

Selling Your Medical Practice

☐ It is wise to use a consultant or valuation expert to handle your sale. Find out what the state law requires and get a copy of the law. _____ _____

Valuing Your Practice

☐ You should seek the advice or assistance of an attorney, accountant, or a professional practice appraiser or valuation expert to help value your practice. There are too many variables to consider (eg, demographics, age of practice, location, condition, replacement cost, and assets) to apply an industry standard estimate. _____ _____

Partnership and Corporate Practices

☐ If you are incorporated or have partners, consult an attorney to review the contract with your partners. _____ _____

Controlled Substances License Termination

☐ Contact the Drug Enforcement Agency (DEA) local office for instructions on the disposal of controlled substances. _____ _____

☐ Void all unused DEA order forms (not to be confused with the state duplicate or triplicate prescription pads) and return them to the DEA or show evidence of shredding. _____ _____

☐ Inform the DEA of your change of address If you want to maintain your DEA registration. _____ _____

☐ If you want to surrender your DEA registration, mail it return-receipt-requested to the DEA, at the appropriate address, along with a letter stating your intent. _____ _____

☐ You can sell the drugs that are not controlled substances. Contact your pharmaceutical representative(s) because pharmaceutical companies may take back unopened, unexpired stock. _____ _____

☐ If selling the drugs is not an option, contact licensed medical relief organizations and donate the items. _____ _____

Check if Completed		Responsible Party	Notes

Controlled Substances (continued)

☐ Be sure to VOID ALL PADS. Ask the DEA and state agency what retention requirements are for your records pertaining to controlled substances when you turn in your registration and duplicate pads.

Informing Your Patients of Your Retirement

☐ Inform your patients of your plans to retire in enough time for them to establish a relationship with a new physician and have copies of their medical records transferred (usually 3–6 months). NOTE: Do not transfer original records, and note the transfer in your retained copy. You may transfer original records if you are retiring and obtain permission from your patients to transfer custody of original records.

☐ Inform patients of move or sale by letter and by publication in local newspapers.

☐ Physicians, their estates, or a physician-custodian should retain medical records (or digital copies) as a safeguard against malpractice liability problems. Ask your malpractice carrier about its requirements.

☐ For patients who made no arrangements for duplication of records at the time of your retirement, you may want to make your attorney the contact person for patients who seek copies of records in the future. You may want to consider scanning your records or placing them in a rented storage location. As a precaution, notify your local medical society of the location of your records.

Insurance Coverage

☐ In advance of your planned retirement date, go over all of your insurance policies with your insurance broker. Request a refund on unexpired policies that are canceled.

☐ Talk to your liability insurance broker about what coverage you will need to protect yourself in retirement.

☐ Be sure that your workers' compensation insurance remains in effect while your employees are still working. Review life, health, and disability policies.

Check if Completed		Responsible Party	Notes

The Office in General

☐ A good office staff makes the practice easier to sell. _____ _____

☐ If you died, would your office staff know what to do? Would they be able to help your family close your practice? Provide them advanced directives. _____ _____

Medical License

☐ If you are retiring or moving, it is important to update your information with your state licensing boards and any credentialing organizations with which you are affiliated. _____ _____

☐ Most states allow you to change your licensure status to Good Standing/Retired. You may also be permitted to renew your medical license at no cost if you request it. Contact your state medical board for details. _____ _____

☐ You may also become exempt from CME requirements by requesting an exemption from the state medical board. _____ _____

Whom to Notify of Your Retirement

☐ *Professional associations:* Your local or state medical society, the American Medical Association (AMA), and your specialty societies. _____ _____

☐ *Major insurance carriers:* These should be advised of your change in status and address due to the long lag time between filing claims and final payments. _____ _____

☐ *Social Security Administration (SSA):* If you are approaching age 65, apply for benefits. Also check with your local medical society for special benefits that it offers. _____ _____

Office Closing List

☐ Notify your patients and arrange for record transmittal and storage. _____ _____

Check if Completed		Responsible Party	Notes
☐	Office insurance, both personnel and contents, must be maintained until business is formally concluded.	_____	_____
☐	File final unemployment return.	_____	_____
☐	Cancel workers' compensation.	_____	_____
☐	Cancel office contents and liabilities when premises are totally vacated.	_____	_____
☐	Keep any accounts receivable coverage until accounts are paid or turned over to a collector.	_____	_____
☐	Professional liability may be canceled only if you plan to stop practicing entirely. If you have been covered under a "claims made" policy, arrange for your "tail" coverage. Be sure to keep all old policies readily accessible.	_____	_____
☐	Notify all suppliers and request final statements. You may be able to return some unopened items for credit.	_____	_____
☐	Notify utilities of the date you want service discontinued.	_____	_____
☐	Check with your accountant. Keep business checking account open for 6 months after closing. This should allow all bills to be paid. Deposits from patients and insurance payments may straggle in after that date but can be deposited to your personal account, as long as a record is kept.	_____	

Items for Your Accountant and Other Advisors

Check if Completed		Responsible Party	Notes
☐	File necessary final tax returns.	_____	_____
☐	Notify the retirement plan of your and your employees' intentions.	_____	_____
☐	Make arrangements for retention of business and personnel records.	_____	_____

Check if Completed		Responsible Party	Notes

Mail Delivery Items

☐ Leave a forwarding address with the post office. Consider renewing it after 6 months to avoid having it expire.   _____   _____

☐ Discontinue magazine subscriptions and ask for a refund or notify printers of your new address.   _____   _____

☐ Write "Retired—Return to Sender" on all "junk mail".   _____   _____

Miscellaneous

☐ Send personal letters of appreciation to individuals who have helped you in your career.   _____   _____

☐ Donate books, journals to a medical library?   _____   _____

☐ Securely store all diplomas, licenses, indications of medical membership.   _____   _____

☐ Give some thought to keeping your answering service active for 3 months to 1 year, depending on local circumstances, your specialty, and/or patient population.   _____   _____

[insert date]

Dear [insert patient name]:

Please be advised that because of my [retirement, reasons of health, or insert other reason], I am discontinuing the practice of medicine on [month] [day], 20[##]. I shall not be able to attend to you professionally after that date.

I suggest that you arrange to place yourself under the care of another physician. If you are not acquainted with another physician, I suggest that you contact the [insert state] Medical Society.

I shall make my records of your case available to the physician you designate. Because the records of your case are confidential, I shall require written authorization to make them available to another physician. At the end of this letter I am including an authorization form. Please complete the form and return it to me.

I am sorry that I cannot continue as your physician. I extend to you my best wishes for your future health and happiness.

Yours very truly,
[insert physician name], MD

To: [insert physician name before mailing to patient], MD

I hereby authorize you to transfer or make available to _____, MD, all of the records and reports relating to my case.

All such documents can be mailed to his/her office address: _____

_____

_____

_____   _____
Patient Signature   Date

Business Office

Solid, organized business practices, whether for a one-person office or a large practice, are essential for success. Obtaining, assembling, and storing correct and complete information about patient visits and about business operations are required. This chapter includes more than 30 forms, checklists, and templates designed to assist in business office operations.

When conducting business with patients and payers, a practice needs a systematic way to obtain, verify, and track financial and payer information. The initial step for a patient's first visit to the practice is patient registration. To make effective use of physician, staff, and patient time, several choices are available for completion of registration forms, such as mailing them to patients for completion before the visit, asking patients to arrive 20 minutes early to complete the forms, and making forms available on a Web site for downloading or on a secure Web site for online completion. If the practice has or plans to have electronic medical records, patients might be asked to complete registration forms on an office computer.

A system is needed to record information when patients or other providers, such as hospital laboratory staff communicating test results, telephone the office. The system needs to include a simple, uniform way to record information and ensure that it is communicated in a timely manner to the appropriate person. In addition, the practice needs to have a sign-in system for patients, which can be simply notifying a receptionist or other staff member in a small practice or a sign-in sheet in larger practices. Provision for maintaining confidentiality of patient information is required. Tools for managing communications with patients and other health care professionals involved in their care are provided in this chapter.

To be paid for services, a medical practice needs to manage relationships with various payers, such as verifying insurance status of patients, obtaining authorization for various procedures, and responding to denials of claims. Clear, accurate, individualized records for each patient encounter are also necessary, not only to support quality and continuity in patient care, but also to receive the proper payment for services. This chapter includes several tools to assist practices in such endeavors.

Tools for a Business Office

Number	Title	Purpose	Notes
03001	Form for a Daily Sign-in Sheet	To keep staff informed about patients who have arrived for appointments	This form can also be used to track patient visits in offices without electronic records.
03002	Template for a New Patient Welcome Letter	To introduce the practice to new patients and inform patients of information needed by the practice	An excellent form letter template to welcome patients to the office and inform them of some of the office's financial policies.
03003	Form for Appointment Scheduling	To assist schedulers in scheduling appointments for realistic time frames that minimize waiting by patients and "downtime" for staff	When this form has been completed by all physicians, physician assistants, and nurse practitioners in the practice, schedulers can use the aggregate data to set up a scheduling grid.
03004	Checklist for Chart Preparation	To identify the needed contents of medical records	In addition to identifying the parts that constitute a medical record, this checklist can be used when evaluating electronic record systems to ensure that all parts of the paper record can be and are included in the electronic record.
03005	Form for a General Patient Information Questionnaire	To obtain patient information as a basis for treatment	Used often in urgent care or for pain medicine clinics.
03006	Form for Patient Registration	To register a patient in a practice	Captures the correct demographic information on each patient.
03007	Form for Patient Responsibility	To inform patients of financial responsibility, the billing process, and terms related to insurance coverage	This is part of the initial patient registration packet.
03008	Form for Patients Rights and Responsibilities	To inform patients of their rights and responsibilities and invite comments about care and treatment	This is part of the initial patient registration packet.
03009	Form for a General Authorization to Release Medical Information	To obtain patients' consent to release confidential medical information	Federal privacy rules prohibit the release of certain confidential information unless specific consent is granted, and such consent is not always a part of a blanket HIPAA privacy release.
03010	Form for a Mail Log	To track the use of postage and disposition of mail and monitor postage costs	The information on this form can be used to help evaluate whether mail is used appropriately and to control postage costs.

Number	Title	Purpose	Notes
03011	Form for Telephone Messages	To record telephone messages	This form is an aid to obtaining proper information during a telephone contact. If one message per page is preferred, one of the two on this form can be deleted.
03012	Form for a Telephone Call Action Chart	To provide guidance for staff about handling telephone calls	This form can be used for training of new office personnel. It also can be used as a basis for a chart for tracking the disposition of telephone calls for quality assurance purposes.
03013	Checklist for Insurance Contracts	To evaluate an insurance contract	A useful tool to compare, contrast and evaluate a commercial contract prior to signing those payor contracts.
03014	Form for a Patient Referral for Specialty Care	To track patient referrals to specialist that are covered by the patient's insurance coverage.	This form can be used to track patient referrals, ensure that consultation reports are received, and identify referral patterns. Using such a form to ensure follow-up can enhance the quality of care and reduce malpractice risks.
03015	Template for a Preappeal Letter Requesting Additional Information	To obtain additional information about denial of a claim submitted for payment	This letter requests information needed by the practice to prepare an appeal about a claim denied because of lack of medical necessity.
03016	Template for a Practice Preauthorization Fax Sheet	To request preauthorization for treatment by fax	Can be set up as a template in MS Word so that it can be filled out by scheduler or hand written and faxed.
03017	Form for Patient Insurance Coverage Verification	To determine a patient's benefits from an insurance company	This form is a great method to capture all the patient insurance coverage that can become a part of the medical record.
03018	Template for a Patient Notification of a Claim Denial	To notify a patient about denial of a claim by the insurance company	This template elicits the patient's support in appealing denial of a claim submitted to a third-party payer.
03019	Template for a Medical-Surgical Predetermination Request	To verify insurance benefits before a procedure is performed	This template can be modified for planned inpatient surgical procedures as well.

Number	Title	Purpose	Notes
03020	Form for Employer-Insurance Verification Information	To verify insurance coverage of patients when employers are self-funded	Verification of benefits for patients who participate in employer self-funded insurance plans must be done through the employee's insurance office.
03021	Template for an Appeal Letter	To appeal denial of a claim submitted to an insurance company	This is an alternative to Tool 03022.
03022	Template for an Appeal Letter to the Payer	To appeal denial of a claim submitted to an insurance company	This letter provides additional information to an insurance carrier about a claim; it may clarify information submitted with the original claim or provide additional supporting rationale for the claim. The letter should be written on the official letterhead of the practice.
03023	Template for a Confirmation of a Claim Denial Rationale to the Payer	To confirm receipt of denial from an insurance company and state objections to the denial	This form assists the physician is writing a request for appeal regarding denials from an insurance carrier because of lack of medical necessity.
03024	Form for Patient Education Opportunities	To ensure adequate patient education about practice and insurer or payer policies.	This multiple-use form can also be used to audit a new hire's grasp of conveying patient information by surveying patients or reviewing charts.
03025	Form for an Encounter (Superbill)	To document the type and level of services provided and the reason	This form is a sample form for documenting services to patients and includes a partial list of procedures and diagnosis codes.
03026	Checklist for Financial Control	To monitor practice revenues	This tool provides the basis for auditing financial practices in the office and can provide guidance for establishing policies and procedures related to cash collections and receipts.
03027	Form for a Medical Record Compliance Evaluation	To assist in audits of documentation in patient records	The findings from audits can be used for quality improvement.
03028	Form for Medication Control	To track medications purchased and used in the practice	This form should be used when performing financial viability audits on cost of medications.

Number	Title	Purpose	Notes
03029	Form for Employees Involved Currently in Patient Test Management Process	To list the employees involved in the patient test management process	Used to meet quality assurance standards for physician office laboratory requirements.
03030	Checklist for Quality Assurance	To provide a list of quality assurance items for an office laboratory	Should be used monthly and quarterly to supervise operations of the quality assurance program in the laboratory.
03031	Template for a Physician Practice Report Card— Staff Productivity Expectations	To evaluate staff productivity in relation to billing, charges, and scheduling follow-up appointments	This form can be used to help the practice set goals for performance related to charges, billing, and follow-up scheduling. The percentage of time each item is done "correctly" should be entered on the form. A means of identifying the actual percentages and comparing them with the expected percentages is needed for meaningful evaluation and for instituting effective improvements when needs are identified.
03032	Form for Controlled Drug Dispensing	To track the use of controlled drugs used on patients while in the office	Controlled substances used in the office on patients during the course of a procedure must be accurately maintained and accounted.
03033	Form for a Controlled Drug Count	To maintain compliance with rules and regulations of the state board of pharmacy and/or the US Drug Enforcement Agency (DEA)	Counting controlled drugs is necessary if the practice stocks narcotics covered by DEA rules. In offices with low-volume use, a weekly, rather than a daily, count may suffice. The drug count record should be kept in a notebook with all drug count records.
03034	Form for a New Patient Census: Monthly and YTD	To indicate growth or lack of growth of the practice. If can also be used to track marketing and promotional responses.	In addition to indicating the numbers of new patients using the practice, this form is used to identify the number of patients no longer using the practice and the reasons. To collect data for this form, a daily or weekly tally should be kept on a similar form to avoid having to check records for an entire month. The monthly tool should be completed on the first working day of the following month, eg, data for January would be recorded on the first working day in February. At the end of a year, data for the year can be compared with data for previous years to identify trends.

Date: _____

Please sign in by printing your complete name and indicating the time that you arrived in the ofice.
NOTE: Because of physician/lab schedules, not all patients will be seen in the order in which they arrive.

	Patient Name	Arrival Time	Control Number [for office use]
1.			
2.			
3.			
4.			
5.			
6.			
7.			
8.			
9.			
10.			
11.			
12.			
13.			
14.			
15.			
16.			
17.			
18.			
19.			
20.			

[Date]

Dear [name of patient],

Thank you for scheduling an appointment with Dr [name] on [day], [date]. It is my pleasure to welcome you to [name of practice] in advance of your first visit.

Following is some information that will help familiarize you with our practice.

[Practice name, address, phone, fax, and Web site address]

Practicing physicians
[insert additional physicians]

Specialty
[insert physicians' specialties]

Business hours
[insert days and appropriate hours]

Contact person
[insert staff name, telephone, and hours available]

Payment policy
It is our payment policy to collect the appropriate payment due from the patient at the time the service is rendered. This may only be your copayment, deductible, and/or coinsurance, but we do ask for payment at the time of your visit. We accept all major credit cards.

Copayment: This is the cost-sharing part of your bill that is a fixed dollar amount designated by your insurance company that is your responsibility to pay at each visit (also known as a copay). Common copayment rates are $10 or $20 per visit, but be aware that copayment rates vary from insurance company to insurance company.

Deductible: This is the amount of cost sharing that you must pay for medical services, often before your health insurance company starts to pay.

Coinsurance: The part of your bill, in addition to a copay, that you must pay. Coinsurance is usually a percentage of the total medical bill—for example 20%.

If you have any questions after reading this information, I will be happy to answer them for you prior to your visit by telephone at [insert telephone number]. Also enclosed are a patient registration form and a privacy form to be completed prior to your scheduled visit. These forms may be faxed to [insert fax number], or you may bring them to your appointment.

Please bring the following information to your visit, if you have not already given it to us prior to your scheduled visit:

Insurance card(s)
Driver's license or other photo identification
Completed patient history form
Completed privacy form

We appreciate your selecting Dr [name] for your medical care and will work hard to serve your needs.

Sincerely,

Appointment Scheduling Guide

_____   _____

Physician Name   Date Form Completed

How much time is required for each visit type?

Visit Type	Time Required
Established Patient	
New Patient	
Consultation	
Physical Examination	
History and Physical	
Blood Pressure Check	
Immunization	

Chart Preparation

In preparing procedure records for the next procedural day, the following checklist will be utilized and included within the record for review by the preoperative nurse prior to the procedure. Any items that have been requested but not received should be identified as such.

Form	Completed and on Chart	N/A	Form	Completed and on Chart	N/A
Summary of Procedures	☐	☐	Pre/Post-Proc Phone Call	☐	☐
Injection Referral Form	☐	☐	Preprocedural Instructions	☐	☐
Patient Demographic Sheet	☐	☐	Physician Order Sheet	☐	☐
HIPAA Privacy Notice	☐	☐	History and Physical	☐	☐
Insurance Card Copies	☐	☐	Informed Consent	☐	☐
Adv. Directives Notification	☐	☐	Pre/Post/Intra-Proc Record	☐	☐
Adv. Directives Document	☐	☐	Discharge Instructions	☐	☐
Operative Report	☐	☐			
Progress Notes	☐	☐			
Anesthesia Record	☐	☐			
Testing, if ordered	☐	☐			
Anesthesia History/Eval	☐	☐			

All forms required to be present on chart for designated procedure are present as indicated.

_____   _____

Signature   Date

Day of Procedure

_____   ☐ N/A (local anesthesia)

The responsible person listed above will remain in the center during the procedure and will drive the patient home from the facility.

Patient Information Questionnaire: General

Confidential Information   Date: _____

The information contained in this questionnaire will be used to help determine the most appropriate medical care required to help you. All information is considered confidential and will not be released unless prior written authorization is given.

Patient's Name: _____

What problems brought you to the office? _____

Have you ever been treated for this condition before?   ☐ Yes   ☐ No

　　If yes, when and by whom? _____

If you are here because of an injury, what were you able to do before without pain, discomfort, or restriction that you are unable to do now? (Check all that apply.)

☐ bend	☐ grip	☐ lie down	☐ sleep	☐ stand up	☐ work at home
☐ reach	☐ walk	☐ drive	☐ lift	☐ sit down	☐ work

☐ other: _____   ☐ other: _____

☐ other: _____   ☐ other: _____

Were you referred to our office for medical care by another physician?   ☐ Yes   ☐ No

　　If so, by whom? _____

Do you have any new complaints or problems since you were referred to our office?   ☐ Yes   ☐ No

　　If yes, explain: _____

Have you been seen by any doctor during the last 3 years?   ☐ Yes   ☐ No

　　If so, doctor's name and specialty? _____
　　　　When were you seen?   From _____ to _____
　　　　What were you seen for? _____

　　If so, doctor's name and specialty? _____
　　　　When were you seen?   From _____ to _____
　　　　What were you seen for? _____

　　If so, doctor's name and specialty? _____
　　　　When were you seen?   From _____ to _____
　　　　What were you seen for? _____

　　If so, doctor's name and specialty? _____
　　　　When were you seen?   From _____ to _____
　　　　What were you seen for? _____

If so, doctor's name and specialty? _____

    When were you seen?   From _____ to _____

    What were you seen for? _____

What medications are you presently taking, if any? _____

_____

_____

Are you now or do you think you may be pregnant?   ☐ Yes   ☐ No

Do you now have or have you ever been treated for cancer or any malignancy?   ☐ Yes   ☐ No

    If yes, when? _____

What allergies do you have? _____

Have you ever had surgery?   ☐ Yes   ☐ No

    If yes, please list the type of surgery and date received:

_____

_____

_____

_____

I certify by my signature that the foregoing information is accurate and truthful to the best of my knowledge.

_____   _____

              Patient Signature   Date

Patient Registration

	New Patient
	Current Patient UPDATE
	Workers' Compensation

Please Complete All

Date / /	Acct No.

Patient Name	Last	First	Initial	Marital Status ☐ S ☐ M ☐ D ☐ W	Sex ☐ M ☐ F

Home Address	City	State	Zip	Home Telephone

Employer/School	Employer/School Address	Work Telephone

Occupation	Social Security Number	Driver's License No. State	Birth Date / /	Age	Living Will? ☐ Yes ☐ No

Spouse or Parent Name	Employer's Address	Work Telephone

Name of Financially Responsible Person (if Different from Patient)	☐ Spouse ☐ Parent ☐ Other

Address (if Different from Patient)	Home Telephone	Work Telephone

Primary Health Insurance Co. Name	Policy Holder	Policy Holder's Relationship to Patient ☐ Self ☐ Spouse ☐ Parent ☐ Other

Insurance Co. Address	ID/Policy No.	Group No.	Coverage Code	Effective Date / /

Secondary Health Insurance Co. Name	Policy Holder	Policy Holder's Relationship to Patient ☐ Self ☐ Spouse ☐ Parent ☐ Other

Insurance Co. Address	ID/Policy No.	Group No.	Coverage Code	Effective Date / /

Family Physician	Referred By	Address	Reference No.	Telephone

Any Member of Family Treated by Our Group Before ☐ Yes ☐ No	Emergency Contact	Telephone

Your Current Problem: Work Related? ☐ Yes ☐ No Accident Case? ☐ Yes ☐ No Automobile Involved? ☐ Yes ☐ No

Have You Missed Time From Work? ☐ No ☐ Yes (specify dates)	If Due to Work-Related Injury, Fill out the Section Below.

Date of Injury / /	Was Injury Reported to Supervisor? ☐ Yes ☐ No	Name of Supervisor

Employer at Time of Injury	Address	Telephone

Description of Injury:

Workers' Compensation Insurance Carrier	Claim Number

Workers' Compensation Insurance Carrier Address	Telephone

Is Attorney Assisting You With This Worker's Comp Claim? ☐ Yes ☐ No

Attorney's Name	Address	Telephone

Patient Responsibility

[insert physician practice logo or letterhead]

Payment Policy

It is our payment policy to collect the appropriate payment due from the patient at the time the service is rendered. This may only be your *copayment or copay*, *deductible*, and/or *coinsurance*, but we do ask for payment at the time of your visit.

- ☐ We have not contacted your health insurance company but anticipate the following payment responsibility.
- ☐ We contacted your health insurance company [insert company name] for an estimate of your health care *benefits* for the following procedures or services:
  [list procedures or services]

Your health insurance company benefit plan identifies that you are responsible for the following estimated charges:

Your insurance company considers the physician to be

☐ *in-network*   ☐ *out-of-network*

$[insert amount]	Deductible
$[insert amount]	Copayment
$[insert amount]	Coinsurance
$[insert amount]	Other charges: [insert type of charge]

- ☐ Your plan policy indicates that a *preadmission approval or certification* is required. The physician office staff received the following authorization number—[insert authorization number]—from your health insurance company.

Patient Medical Billing Process

The physician office staff, as a courtesy to you, will submit a medical bill to your *primary health insurance company* for processing. It is important to give your updated information to the physician office staff, since your complete and current information is necessary to submit an accurate *claim form* to your insurance company. The remaining claim will be sent to a *secondary health insurance company*, if provided, after the payment is received from the primary health insurance company.

The physician office staff will mail to you a *bill/invoice/statement* that contains the total cost of your service(s) and/or procedure(s) received during your office visit. You may expect this bill within _____ days. The health insurance company payment will be deducted from the bill when it is received by the office staff.

You are responsible for any outstanding balance, such as *noncovered charges*, as outlined in your health insurance company policy. These charges are listed on the *advance medical services payment agreement* or *advanced beneficiary notice (ABN)*.

Patient Glossary of Terms

Advance medical services payment agreement—If your health insurance company will not pay for a procedure or service, the physician or hospital will request you review and sign an advance medical services payment agreement. This notice will assist you in determining whether you want to have the procedure or service performed and how you prefer to pay for it.

Advanced beneficiary notice (ABN)—If Medicare will not pay for a procedure or service, the physician or hospital will request you to review and sign an advanced beneficiary notice. This notice will assist you in determining whether you want to have the procedure or service performed and how you prefer to pay for it.

Benefit—The amount your plan will pay a physician, group, or hospital as stated in your policy, toward the cost of the service or procedure to be performed by the physician.

Bill/invoice/statement—The summary of your medical bill.

Claim—The form that the physician files with a health insurance company that details the services and procedures performed by the physician, on your behalf, and other pertinent data that are required by the health insurance company to receive payment.

Copayment or copay—The part of your medical bill you must pay each time you visit the doctor. This is a preset fee determined by your health insurance policy.

Coinsurance—The part of your bill, in addition to a copay, that you must pay. Coinsurance is usually a percentage of the total medical bill, for example, 20%.

Deductible—The amount you must pay for medical treatment before your health insurance company starts to pay, for example, $500 per individual or $1500 per family. In most cases, a new deductible must be satisfied each calendar year.

In-network—The physician has contracted a payment schedule with the health insurance company to provide you with medical care. The physician will submit your medical bill directly to the health insurance company for payment. However, you may be responsible for a copayment, deductible, and/or coinsurance according to your health insurance company benefit plan.

Noncovered charges—Costs for medical treatment that your health insurance company does not pay. You may want to determine whether your treatment is covered by your health insurance policy before you are billed for these charges by the doctor's office.

Out-of-network—The physician is not contracted with the health insurance company to provide you with medical treatment. You are responsible for the payment for the medical care. The physician may agree to submit your medical bill directly to the payer for payment. However, you may be responsible for an increased copayment, deductible, coinsurance, and/or additional charges according to your insurance company benefit plan.

Preadmission approval or certification number—A number authorizing the health insurance company to pay benefits for your care. You may need to obtain an approval number from your health insurance representative before you see the doctor in order for the health insurance company to pay for your medical treatment. Your doctor's office staff might be able to help you obtain the approval from the health insurance company.

Primary health insurance company—The health insurance company that is responsible to pay your benefits first when you have more than one health insurance plan.

Secondary health insurance company—The secondary health insurance company is not the first payer of your claims. The remaining claim balance will be sent to a secondary health insurance company, if provided, after payment is received from the primary health insurance company.

For questions about your bill, please call [contact name] at [telephone number] Monday through Friday between the hours of [beginning time] and [ending time].

Patient's Name (Please Print)_____

Patient's Signature_____

Date_____

Patient Rights and Responsibilities

Patient Rights

1. You have the right to dignified and respectful care.
2. You have the right to know about and understand your physical condition.
3. You have the right to obtain any information requested by you to give informed consent before any treatment and/or procedure.
4. You have the right, at your own expense, to consult with another physician or specialist.
5. You have the right to refuse treatment, as permitted by law, and to be informed of the consequences of your refusal.
6. You have the right to be treated in a safe environment that is free of physical and psychological threats.
7. You have the right to privacy regarding visitors, mail, and/or telephone conversations.
8. You have the right to expect that all communications and records regarding your care will be held confidential.
9. You have the right to expect continuity of care and that you will not be discharged or transferred to another facility without prior notice.
10. You have the right to communicate verbally or in writing with anyone outside the practice and to expect that an interpreter will be provided if language is a barrier.
11. You have the right to know the identity, professional status, and institutional affiliation of anyone treating you.
12. You have the right to request an itemized statement of all services provided to you through this practice.
13. You have the right to be informed of all practice rules and regulations governing your conduct as a patient and to understand the procedure for registering a complaint.
14. You have the right to treatment or accommodations required by your medical condition regardless of race, creed, sex, or national origin.

Patient Responsibilities

1. You are responsible for providing complete information about your health and for reporting the effects of your treatment.
2. You will be responsible for participating in the development of your plan of care.
3. You will be responsible for attending scheduled therapy and participating in activities prescribed by your treatment plan.
4. You will be responsible for considering the rights of other patients and office personnel during your treatment in this practice.
5. You are responsible for following practice rules and regulations.

Concern/Complaint Procedure

We want to hear from you if you have any concerns, complaints, or compliments regarding your stay treatment and care in our practice. Please inform any staff member.

Response to a concern/complaint will take place within 24 hours. Concerns/complaints will be monitored and the information utilized to improve our program.

I have been made aware of my rights and responsibilities and the concern/complaint procedure.

Date:_____   Patient: _____

Caregiver and relationship: _____

Witness: _____

Witness: _____
        (if patient is unable to document signature, two persons must be witness)

Authorization to Release Medical Information

I AUTHORIZE: TO RELEASE TO:

_____   _____
Name of sending person/organization   Name of receiving person/organization

_____   _____
Street Address   Street Address

_____   _____
City   State   Zip Code   City   State   Zip Code

Patient's Signature: _____

INFORMATION TO BE RELEASED: (Check all applicable)

☐ All Information   ☐ All Progress Notes   ☐ Lab Reports   ☐ X-Ray Reports

☐ Electrocardiogram (EKG)   ☐ Allergy Records   ☐ Immunization Records   ☐ Other: _____

SPECIAL AUTHORIZATION: (check all that are applicable and sign below)

By signing below, you are authorizing the office to release any and all information regarding:

☐ Alcohol   ☐ Drugs   ☐ Mental Health   ☐ Sexually Transmitted Diseases   ☐ HIV   ☐ AIDS

Signature:

If this release pertains to alcohol, drug, or mental health information, please note that this information has been disclosed to you from records protected by federal confidentiality rules (42 CFR part 2). The federal rules prohibit you from making any further disclosure of this information unless additional further disclosure is expressly permitted by written consent of the person to whom it pertains or as otherwise permitted by 42 CFR part 2. A general authorization for the release of medical or other information is not sufficient for this purpose. The federal rules restrict any use of the information to criminally investigate or prosecute any alcohol or drug abuse patient.

RECORDS FROM THE PERIOD: _____/_____/_____ to _____/_____/_____

PURPOSE OR NEED FOR DISCLOSURE: (Check applicable purpose)

☐ Continued Medical Care   ☐ Payment of Insurance Claim   ☐ Legal

☐ Personal   ☐ Workers' Compensation Claim   ☐ Other: _____

I understand that this authorization shall be valid for one year. I understand that I may revoke this consent at any time except to the extent that action has already been taken.

I understand that a reasonable fee may be charged for duplication of records. An estimate of those charges will be provided upon request prior to duplication.

The requestor may be provided with a copy of this authorization.

Mail Log

Date:

Sender's Name	Patient's Name	Type of Mail

Telephone Message

Date: ____/____/____   Time: _____   Taken by: _____

Person Calling: _____

□ Medical Record Attached   □ Billing Account Attached

Physician's Name: _____

re: Patient _____

□ HOLDING   Call At: □ ASAP   □ Noon   □ 5:00 P.M.

□ Personal   □ Financial   □ Medical concern

Insurance claim issue: □ NO   □ YES/Claim Number: _____

Date of service: _____

Medical action needed: _____

_____

□ Prescription refill   Detail: _____

□ Lab result(s): _____

□ Reference request for: _____

Telephone number: _____

Remarks: _____

_____

_____

Symptoms

□ Bleeding*

□ Cough

□ Dizziness

□ Drug reaction*

□ Fever: _____ °

□ General discomfort

□ Hysterical*

□ Incoherent*

□ Injury*

□ Itching

□ Pain*

□ Rash

□ Swelling

□ Unconscious*

□ Weak

□ Other (explain in remarks section)

If severe, place patient on HOLD. Relay to Physician IMMEDIATELY.

Telephone Message

Date: ____/____/____   Time: _____   Taken by: _____

Person Calling: _____

□ Medical Record Attached   □ Billing Account Attached

Physician's Name: _____

re: Patient _____

□ HOLDING   Call At: □ ASAP   □ Noon   □ 5:00 P.M.

□ Personal   □ Financial   □ Medical concern

Insurance claim issue: □ NO   □ YES/Claim Number: _____

Date of service: _____

Medical action needed: _____

_____

□ Prescription refill   Detail: _____

□ Lab result(s): _____

□ Reference request for: _____

Telephone number: _____

Remarks: _____

_____

_____

Symptoms

□ Bleeding*

□ Cough

□ Dizziness

□ Drug reaction*

□ Fever: _____ °

□ General discomfort

□ Hysterical*

□ Incoherent*

□ Injury*

□ Itching

□ Pain*

□ Rash

□ Swelling

□ Unconscious*

□ Weak

□ Other (explain in remarks section)

If severe, place patient on HOLD. Relay to Physician IMMEDIATELY.

Telephone Call Action Chart

Refer to the office telephone matrix (includes the specifics for each physician), but policies in general are as follows:

Refer to Physician at Once

- Emergency
- Very ill patient who is currently under treatment
- Request for consultation
- Referral call from another physician
- Personal call from another physician

Refer to the Nurse

- Request for test information by patient

Take Message, Call Will Be Returned

- Request for information from patient's family
- Pharmacist for prescription renewal
- Pharmacist for new prescription
- Business calls for physician

Receptionist Should Handle

- Request for appointments, if applicable
- Salespersons—make appointments

Billing Personnel Should Handle

- Request for information from insurance company
- Request for insurance information
- Calls about accounts receivable

Note: Telephone messages or instruction provided to patients should *always* be noted in the medical chart.

Insurance Contracts

Check if Completed		Responsible Party	Notes
☐	All attachments, addenda, and documents referenced are attached.	_____	_____
☐	All verbal representations made to you are referenced in writing.	_____	_____
☐	The contract adequately identifies the entities responsible for payment and provides all contact information needed.	_____	_____
☐	You have confirmed the information by actual contact.	_____	_____
☐	You have spoken with other physicians or administrators experienced with the plan and asked about ease of communication, prompt payment, and hassle factors.	_____	_____
☐	You have requested and obtained a financial statement or other support information verifying the plan's solvency and financial strength.	_____	_____
☐	You have obtained verification that the plan has stop-loss coverage and liability insurance.	_____	_____
☐	The contract indicates that your claims will be paid within a certain number of days, and it contains an incentive for the payer to comply, such as interest or penalties.	_____	_____
☐	The contract specifies the reimbursement rate in dollars for at least some procedures or the capitation rate per member per month.	_____	_____
☐	The contract allows a reasonable time to submit claims and has a provision for extension of that time because of unforeseen circumstances (for example, employee termination or fraud, severe weather, computer malfunction).	_____	_____
☐	The contract has a claims appeal process, and you have checked references to find out how well it works.	_____	_____
☐	The contract does not require you to hold the plan harmless or indemnify it for any actions other than your own.	_____	_____

Check if Completed		Responsible Party	Notes
☐	The contract does not require you to pay the plan's legal fees in a patient action, dispute, or for any other reason.	_____	_____
☐	The contract says you will be compensated for any extra activities required (such as quality assurance or utilization review) and you will receive adequate insurance for those activities.	_____	_____
☐	The contract adequately describes quality assurance, utilization review, dispute resolution, and other oversight functions. Those functions appear to be fair, and physicians other than those administratively employed by the plan have input.	_____	_____
☐	The contract does not hold you to a standard higher than "a reasonable physician acting under the same or similar situation."	_____	_____
☐	The contract does not require you to obtain an unreasonable amount of professional liability insurance or other coverage. It also does not require that your policy cover the insurer.	_____	_____
☐	The contract does not prohibit you from participating in other plans.	_____	_____
☐	The contract does not allow your name to be used in marketing activities without your consent.	_____	_____
☐	There is a confidentiality clause prohibiting the plan from making disclosures about you that are not indicated in the contract.	_____	_____
☐	The contract does not require you to significantly change your billing practices or use of staff, alter your hours, or otherwise make major changes in the way you practice.	_____	_____
☐	The contract provides an adequate panel of specialists and ancillary services.	_____	_____
☐	The contract allows you to stop taking new patients without penalty.	_____	_____
☐	The contract allows you to bill patients your normal fee for noncovered services and medically unnecessary services demanded by patients and for charges the plan is unable to pay or fails to pay.	_____	_____

Check if Completed		Responsible Party	Notes
☐	The contract provides explicit instructions on verification of patients' eligibility.	_____	_____
☐	The contract provides for reimbursement when the insurer mistakenly indicates a patient is eligible under its plan.	_____	_____
☐	Adequate patients or lives will be available to you from the plan.	_____	_____
☐	If capitated, you will receive fee-for-service until an appropriate number of lives are provided.	_____	_____
☐	If capitated, you are (ideally) capitated differently for each demographic group you will treat.	_____	_____
☐	If capitated, the services included are clearly defined.	_____	_____
☐	The contract allows you an "easy out" in case of dispute, inadequate patient volume, or any other reason, without penalty and within a reasonable period.	_____	_____

Patient Referral for Specialty Care

					Report	
Referral Name	**Date**	**Patient's Name**	**HMO/MCO**	**Specialist**	**Date Due**	**Date Received**

[Date]

Attn: [name]
Provider Appeals Department
[Address]
[City, State ZIP code]

Dear [director of claims/medical director]:

On [date denial letter received], I received a letter from [name/title of sender] stating [treatment/service] was denied for [patient name] because of lack of medical necessity.

The American Medical Association (AMA) defines *medical necessity* as "health care services or products that a prudent physician would provide to a patient for the purpose of preventing, diagnosing, or treating an illness, injury, disease, or its symptoms in a manner that is (a) in accordance with the generally accepted standards of medical practice; (b) clinically appropriate in terms of type, frequency, extent, site, and duration; and (c) not primarily for the convenience of the patient, treating physician, or other health care provider."

We request that [payer] use the AMA definition of medical necessity when making determinations on medically necessary treatments and/or health care services.

The accompanying explanation of benefits did not provide adequate information to support this denial; therefore, I am requesting the following information: [list requested information].

Please furnish the source and content of the information on which the medical necessity denial decision was based. Also, please provide a description of the information necessary for approval of the treatment/service.

We also would appreciate copies of any expert medical opinions that have been secured by your company about treatment/service of this nature and its efficacy so the treating physician may respond to its applicability to this patient's condition.

Thank you for your assistance.

Sincerely,

[patient accounts manager]

cc: [patient name]

Request for Preauthorization Fax Sheet

To _____ Fax _____

From _____ Phone _____ Fax _____

Number of pages sent (including cover page) _____

If you have any problems with this transmittal, please contact [insert name] at [insert telephone number].

Re: **Preauthorization request**

Health plan member name: [insert member name]
Patient name: [insert name]
Patient health plan identification number (policy number): [insert number]
Group number: [insert group number]
Examining physician: [insert physician's name]
Examination date: [insert date]

We are requesting your expedited review for the preauthorization of the following procedures and/or services for the above-mentioned patient. The above-named physician, as a result of the evaluation on [insert date] has evaluated the patient and recommended the following procedures and/or services.

Procedure: [insert procedure]
CPT code: [insert code]
Practice fee schedule amount: [insert amount]
Total amount: [insert total]

We request your assignment of preauthorization for the above-listed procedures and/or services. Please fax the completed information consisting of the following:

- Assigned preauthorization number for all of the listed procedures and/or services
- Listing of any nonauthorized procedures and/or services with supporting rationale
- Any presurgical requirements of the health plan that must be met prior to delivery of services to the patient

If you require any additional information, please contact [insert name] at [insert telephone number] between the hours of [insert beginning time] and [insert ending time].

Preauthorization form

Please complete the following information and fax to [insert name] at [insert fax number].

Name of authorizing representative for health plan _____

Telephone number for authorizing representative _____

Preauthorization number _____

Comments or requirements _____

_____

_____

Date: _____ Practice: _____ Verification By: _____

Patient Name: _____ Account #: _____

Date of Birth: _____ Social Security #: _____

Employer: _____ Phone/Contact: _____

Accident Date: _____ Accident Location: _____

Patient Care Plan

Dx 1: _____ Dx 2: _____

Dx 3: _____ Dx 4: _____

Patient Care Plans/Services: _____

Insurance Data

Insurance 1 (Primary)

Billing Address: _____

Insurance Contact Name: _____ Telephone: _____

Policy #: _____ Plan #: _____ Group #: _____

Coverage Effective Dates From: _____ To: _____

Policyholder: _____ Relationship: _____

Insurance 2 (Secondary)

Billing Address: _____

Insurance Contact Name: _____ Telephone: _____

Policy #: _____ Plan #: _____ Group #: _____

Coverage Effective Dates From: _____ To: _____

Policyholder: _____ Relationship: _____

Basic Benefits	Primary	Secondary
1. Preexisting wait period		
2. Annual deductible amount	$	$
3. Deductible paid to date	$	$
4. Out-of-pocket expenses		
a. Coinsurance ($ or %)		
b. Copayment @ TOS	$	$
5. Calendar year maximum	$ / days	$ / days
6. Lifetime maximum	$ / days	$ / days
7. Remaining benefits	$ / days	$ / days
8. Medical records required?	☐ yes ☐ no	☐ yes ☐ no
9. Coordinate benefits (x-over)?	☐ yes ☐ no	☐ yes ☐ no
10. Second opinion requirements?	☐ yes ☐ no	☐ yes ☐ no
11. Verified with (name)		
12. Phone number of above		
13. Date verified		

Procedures and Services	Covered?	Coverage Details/Limits
Office services	☐ yes ☐ no	
Hospital	☐ yes ☐ no	
Consultations	☐ yes ☐ no	
Emergency department visits	☐ yes ☐ no	
Laboratory (Chem)	☐ yes ☐ no	
Procedures	☐ yes ☐ no	
Injections/treatments	☐ yes ☐ no	
Supplies	☐ yes ☐ no	
Drugs/medications	☐ yes ☐ no	
Exclusions		

[date]

[Mr/Mrs/Ms] [name]
[address]
[city, state ZIP code]

Dear [patient name],

This letter is being sent to notify you that your health insurance company denied the following service [procedure name] that was provided to you on [date].

Our office filed an appeal challenging your health insurance company's position, and we are requesting that the claim be reconsidered for payment. A copy of the appeal letter is enclosed for your reference.

Although our office will follow up on the status of the appeal, we request that you contact your health insurance company regarding this matter. Our experience has proven that health insurance companies are most responsive to the patient's request. By contacting the health insurance company, you will help expedite the review process as well as increase the likelihood of claim payment. If your health insurance company refuses to issue payment despite our appeal efforts, you may need to pursue the matter further with assistance from your company's benefits department and/or state insurance commissioner's office.

We appreciate your cooperation through this appeal process. Should you have any questions, please contact [staff name/department] at [telephone number].

Sincerely,

[practice contact name/department]

enclosure

[Health plan]
Attn: Medical Predetermination
[Address]
[City, State ZIP code]

Re: **Predetermination request**

Patient name: [insert name]
Health plan member name: [insert member name]
Patient health plan identification number (policy number): [insert number]
Group number: [insert group number]
Examining physician: [insert physician's name]
Examination date: [insert date]

To whom it may concern:

The following information is being provided to predetermine surgical benefits for an outpatient surgical procedure. Outlined below are the procedural and diagnostic codes, description, and cost for the recommended surgery. Copies of applicable medical records are included to support the medical necessity of the procedure.

CPT codes	ICD-9-CM codes

Description of procedure/service

Fees

The following information provides a brief summary of the patient's chief complaints and history of present illness:

Please be advised that the above named patient has been under [physician name]'s care since [date] for [insert summary of complaints and illness history].

Please provide our practice with written notification regarding benefit coverage upon determination of this case. Should additional information be needed, please contact our practice at [insert telephone number].

Sincerely,

[physician name and/or practice manager name]

Enclosures

Patient Name: _____

Date: _____

Employer Name: _____

Employer Address: _____

Benefits Coordinator: _____ Telephone Number: _____

Insurance Carrier: _____ Plan Name: _____

Policy #: _____ Plan #: _____ Group #: _____

Type of Plan: □ Traditional   □ 80/20   □ HMO   □ PPO   □ Other: _____

Mail Insurance Forms to: □ Carrier   □ Employer

Billing Address: _____

Contact Person: _____ Telephone Number: _____

Renewal Period – Medical Benefits and Limits Are Renewed on (M/D/Y): (Date): _____

E-mail Address: _____

Basic Coverage

Physician Payment Schedule: □ UCR   □ RBRVS   □ Other Data: _____

Percentage of COB (eg, 80/20): _____% Insurance Coverage _____ % Patient Copayment

Annual Outpatient Deductible: _____ Amount of Deductible Remaining: _____

Maximum Benefit: _____

Noncovered Services: _____

Diagnostic Benefits

Percentage of COB (eg, 80/20): _____% Insurance Coverage _____ % Patient Copayment

Annual Outpatient Deductible: _____ Amount of Deductible Remaining: _____

Maximum Benefit: _____

Noncovered Services: _____

Major Medical Coverage

Annual Outpatient Deductible: _____

Amount of Deductible Remaining: _____

Maximum Benefit: _____

Noncovered Services: _____

Form Used: □ Company-Specific Form   □ CMS-1500   □ Other: _____

Notes: _____

_____

[date]

Attn: [name]
Provider Appeals Department
[address]
[city, state ZIP code]

Re:

Policyholder's (ie, Subscriber's) name: [insert name]
Health plan identification number: [insert identification number]
Group number: [insert group number]
Patient name: [insert patient name]
Claim number: [insert claim number]
Submission date: [insert date]
Treating physician: [insert physician's name]
Physician or group identification number: [insert number]

Dear [Madam or Sir]:

We are appealing your decision and request reconsideration of the attached claim that you denied on [date].

We feel these services should be allowed and reimbursed for the following reason(s):
     [insert reasons]

Thank you for reviewing and reversing this claims denial. If you require any additional information, please contact [staff name] at [telephone number] between the hours of [insert time that staff is available to answer calls, eg, 8:00 AM to 5:00 PM].

A copy of your explanation of benefits/remittance advice and the initially submitted CMS-1500 form is enclosed.

Sincerely,

[physician name]
[identification number]

Enclosures

[date]

Attn: [name]
Provider Appeals Department
[address]
[city, state ZIP code]

Re: Claim denial

Insured/plan member: [insert insured/plan member]
Payer identification number: [insert payer identification number]
Group number: [insert group number]
Patient name: [insert patient name]
Claim number: [insert claim number]
Claim date: [insert claim date]

Dear [Mr/Mrs] [name]:

We are appealing your decision and request reconsideration of the attached claim that you denied on [date].

We feel these charges should be allowed for the following reason(s):
        [insert reasons]

Thank you for reviewing and reversing this claim denial. If you require any additional information, please contact [staff name] at [telephone number] between the hours of [insert time that staff is available to answer calls, eg, 8:00 AM to 5:00 PM].

Sincerely,

[physician name]
[identification name]

Enclosure

[date]

Attn: [name]
Provider Appeals Department
[address]
[city, state ZIP code]

Re: Medical necessity denial

Insured/plan member: [insert insured/plan member]
Payer identification number: [insert payer identification number]
Group number: [insert group number]
Patient name: [insert patient name]
Claim number: [insert claim number]
Claim date: [insert claim date]

Dear [Mr/Mrs] [name]:

This letter confirms our conversation today about the care of [patient name] and requests a review of this clinically inappropriate denial. As a physician, I have an ethical and legal duty to advocate for any care I believe will materially benefit my patients. As you will recall, I recommended [describe procedure, course of treatment, referral, etc], which I believe is medically necessary for the following reasons: [reason procedure or service will be performed].

[Payer] has made a decision to deny this care. I will inform the patient in writing of this decision, including the alternative treatment options: [list alternative treatment options]. In addition, I will include this letter as part of the patient's medical record.

If this is not accurate, please advise me promptly. Again, I believe this [procedure, test, course of treatment] is medically necessary. In my clinical judgment the [plan]'s denial of coverage is not in the best interest of the patient.

In the event that [patient name], the family, or an employer wishes to hear your reasoning, I will refer them directly to you to avoid any misrepresentation.

Sincerely,

[Physician name]

cc: [patient name]

Opportunities for Staff to Educate Patients about Financial Policies Audit Form

Column 1: Preregistration/appointment scheduling *(patient education opportunity #1)*
Column 2: Practice Web site *(patient education opportunity #2)*
Column 3: Welcome letter *(patient education opportunity #3)*
Column 4: Insurance verification *(patient education opportunity #4)*
Column 5: Appointment reminder *(patient education opportunity #5)*
Column 6: Patient check-in *(patient education opportunity #6)*
Column 7: Patient checkout *(patient education opportunity #7)*
Column 8: Claim processing/patient invoice/claim collections *(patient education opportunity #8)*
Column 9: Physician appeal letter *(patient education opportunity #9)*

	1	2	3	4	5	6	7	8	9
Identify whether the patient is new, existing, or a referral	X				X	X			
Identify the specific reason for the patient visit	X	X			X	X			
Record the patient's full name as it is spelled on his/her insurance card	X				X	X			
Gather the general patient registration information, such as the patient's demographics and payer information	X	X							
Complete insurance verification				X					
Schedule a convenient appointment time for the patient and physician	X	X					X		
Collect the patient's contact information and his/her preferred place of contact	X	X				X	X		
Review the practice's payment policy	X	X	X		X	X	X		
Indicate which credit cards are accepted by the practice	X	X	X		X	X	X		
Collect or remind the patient of any outstanding balance	X	X			X	X	X		
Inform the patient that, at the time of the visit, he/she should bring in an updated insurance card and driver's license or another type of photo identification	X	X	X		X				
Collect and record the referring physician's contact information, if appropriate	X	X							
Remind the patient that the referral authorization, records (eg, child's immunization record) and/or test results should be available at the time of the visit	X	X	X		X				
Remind the patient to bring in all current medications at the time of the visit	X	X	X		X				
Request that the patient complete the history form that will be placed in the mail or provide the Web site where the patient can download the form prior to the visit	X	X	X			X			
Identify any additional practice policies (eg, prescription refills)	X	X	X		X	X			
Provide the patient with a contact number to use if the patient is unable to make the scheduled visit or has additional administrative and clinical questions	X	X	X		X		X		
Provide a list of physicians' names and specialties		X	X						
Indicate the practice's hours and holiday schedule		X	X						
Provide a list of hospitals with which the physician is affiliated		X	X						
Provide the practice's Web site address for additional resources	X		X		X				

	1	2	3	4	5	6	7	8	9
Provide a list of payers and the associated products (eg, PPO, POS, HMO) that the physician accepts		X	X						
Confirm the date and time of the scheduled patient visit			X		X				
Verify whether there has been any change in the patient's health insurance information (for a returning or established patient)						X			
Request any missing or correct any incorrect patient information						X			
Make a copy of the patient's health insurance card						X			
Explain and distribute the practice's payment and privacy policies						X			
Explain and receive a signed acknowledgment from the patient that should include the practice's policies on patient billing, primary and secondary payer processing, and patient payment expectations						X			
Explain when and how test results will be communicated to the patient and receive a signed waiver that indicates whether the patient gives permission for leaving test results on an answering machine or in voice mail						X	X		
Provide a physician referral form, obtain an authorization (if required by payer), and advise the patient if the referred physician is considered out-of-network by his/her payer							X		
Explain and collect the patient's copayment and/or deductible, if not collected during the check-in process						X	X		
Explain and complete the patient responsibility sheet							X		
Determine and agree upon a payment plan with the patient if the patient indicates he/she is unable to make a payment for the procedures and/or services provided							X		
Explain the claim processing/patient invoice/claim collections processes								X	
Copy the patient on the initial medical necessity appeal letter that requests the rationale for the denial by the payer									X
Send a follow-up appeal letter that contains the clinical support for the procedure or service in response to the payer's stated rationale									X
Send a notification letter to the patient requesting his/her involvement									X
Send a confirmation follow-up appeal letter to the payer with the adverse decision clearly stated and copy the patient									X

[insert physician name]
[insert physician specialty]
[insert office address]
[insert city, state ZIP code]

Telephone: [insert number]

			DATE	
LAST NAME FIRST	ACCOUNT #	DOB	☐ Male ☐ Female	
INSURANCE	PLAN #	SUBSCRIBER #	GROUP #	

OFFICE CARE

	DESCRIPTION	CPT-MOD		
	NEW PATIENT			
	Focused	99201		
	Expanded	99202		
	Detailed	99203		
	Comprehensive–Mod.	99204		
	Comprehensive–High	99205		
	ESTABLISHED PATIENT			
	Minimal	99211		
	Focused	99212		
	Expanded	99213		
	Detailed	99214		
	Comprehensive–Mod.	99215		
	Comprehensive–High	99216		
	CONSULTATION OFFICE			
	Focused	99241		
	Expanded	99242		
	Detailed	99243		
	Comprehensive–Mod.	99254		
	Comprehensive–High	99265		
	Dr.			
	Post-op exam	99024		
	EVALUATION/MANAGEMENT			
	Brief–30 minutes	99361		
	Intermediate–60	99362		
	Telephone–Brief	99371		
	Telephone–Intermed.	99372		
	Telephone–Complex	99373		

PROCEDURES

DESCRIPTION	CPT-MOD		
Treadmill	93015		
24-hr Holter	93224		
Recording only	93225		
Interp. & report	93227		
EKG and interp.	93000		
EKG (Medicare)	93005		
Sigmoidscopy	45300		
Sigmoidscopy (flex)	45330		
Sigmoid (flex) w/bx	45331		

DIAGNOSIS CODES

052.9	Chickenpox, NOS	266.2	B12 deficiency w/o anemia	309.9	Adjustment reaction, unspecified
111.9	Dermatomycosis, unspecified	276.5	Dehydration	305.00	Alcohol abuse, unspecified
009.1	Gastroenteritis, infectious	250.91	Diabetes mellitus, I, compl	303.90	Alcoholism, unspecified
007.1	Giardiasis	250.01	Diabetes mellitus, I, uncompl	331.0	Alzheimer's
098.0	Gonorrhea, acute, lower GU	250.90	Diabetes mellitus, II, compl	307.1	Anorexia nervosa
054.9	Herpes simplex, any site	250.00	Diabetes mellitus, II, uncompl	300.00	Anxiety state, unspecified
053.9	Herpes zoster, NOS	250.13	Diabetic ketoacidosis	314.01	Attention deficit, w/ hyperactivity
042	HIV Disease	271.9	Glucose intolerance	314.00	Attention deficit, w/o hyperactivity
V08	HIV positive, asymp	240.9	Goiter, unspecified	307.51	Bulimia
136.9	Infectious/parasitic dis unspec	274.9	Gout, unspecified	312.90	Conduct disorder, unspecified
487.1	Influenza w/ upper resp sx	275.42	Hypercalcemia	311	Depressive disorder, NOS
007.9	Intestinal protozoa, NOS	276.7	Hyperkalemia	305.90	Drug abuse, unspecified
088.81	Lyme disease	276.0	Hypernatremia		
055.9	Measles, NOS	252.0	Hyperparathyroidism		

DIAGNOSIS				
RETURN APPOINTMENT	REFERRING MD	SIGNATURE		☐ Cash ☐ Check ☐ Credit

Financial Control

Check if Completed		Responsible Party	Notes

Cash Collections and Receipts

☐ Is a change fund being maintained? _____ _____

☐ Are receipts issued for cash payments? _____ _____

☐ Are receipts prenumbered? _____ _____

☐ Are carbon copies of receipts kept? _____ _____

☐ Are payments received indicated as check or cash on the receipts and daysheets/ computer run? _____ _____

☐ Is cash totaled daily to agree with daysheets/computer run? _____ _____

☐ Are damaged receipts voided and left in the book attached to daysheet? _____ _____

☐ Are employees who handle cash bonded? _____ _____

Deposits

☐ Is deposit prepared daily? _____ _____

☐ Are deposits held overnight stored safely? _____ _____

☐ Are the carbon copy deposit slips attached to the daysheet/computer run? _____ _____

☐ Is the bank statement opened only by the physician or accountant? _____ _____

☐ Is the bank statement mailed to the physician's home? _____ _____

☐ Does amount deposited to business account from receipts balance with month-end totals? _____ _____

Daysheets and Financial Cards

☐ If on a manual/pegboard system, are they used correctly? _____ _____

☐ Is there an individual daysheet/computer run for each day? _____ _____

Check if Completed		Responsible Party	Notes

Daysheets and Financial Cards (continued)

☐   Does the physician review and initial the daysheets/computer run?

☐   Are daysheets/daily computer runs compared with appointment book and financial records monthly?

☐   Are all accounts with balances billed, even those pending insurance?

If manual:

☐   Are daysheets and financial cards prepared in ink?

☐   Is a tape of accounts receivable cards run at the end of each month and balanced with A/R on daysheets?

☐   Are financial cards stored safely?

☐   Are all financial cards returned to card files nightly?

If computerized:

☐   When possible, are billing and collection duties done by separate persons?

☐   Is backup on the computer performed daily?

☐   Are disks stored off-site in a safe place?

Petty Cash

☐   Are cash expenditures itemized?

☐   Are receipts kept for petty cash expenditures?

☐   Is a running balance kept of petty cash?

☐   Does the cash balance agree with the records?

☐   Is it balanced monthly?

☐   Are employees' personal belongings kept away from front-office area?

Check if Completed		Responsible Party	Notes

Employees

☐   Are employees required to rotate duties and responsibilities?   _____   _____

☐   Are refund checks approved by the physician?_____   _____

☐   Does the physician review write-offs and adjustments monthly?   _____   _____

☐   Are accounts in internal collection contacted at least monthly?   _____   _____

Accounts Payable and Miscellaneous

☐   Does the physician sign all checks?   _____   _____

☐   Does the physician refrain from keeping a signature stamp in the office?   _____   _____

☐   Does the physician refrain from "skimming" or "dipping" into the petty cash?   _____   _____

☐   Does a CPA or other outside person perform periodic reviews?   _____   _____

Medical Record Compliance Evaluation

Site Address: _____

Report Received By: _____

Physician Name: _____ ID No.: _____

Specialty: _____ Evaluator: _____

PT ID: _____

Date: ___/___/___ Signature: _____

	Patient ID No.	Patient ID No.	Patient ID No.	Patient ID No.	Patient ID No.	Patient ID No.
Are adverse reactions and allergies noted and flagged?	Yes No NA	Yes No NA	Yes No NA	Yes No NA	Yes No NA	Yes No NA
Are all entries dated?	Yes No NA	Yes No NA	Yes No NA	Yes No NA	Yes No NA	Yes No NA
Are all entries legible?	Yes No NA	Yes No NA	Yes No NA	Yes No NA	Yes No NA	Yes No NA
Are all entries signed?	Yes No NA	Yes No NA	Yes No NA	Yes No NA	Yes No NA	Yes No NA
Are preventive services being utilized?	Yes No NA	Yes No NA	Yes No NA	Yes No NA	Yes No NA	Yes No NA
Are problems from previous visits addressed?	Yes No NA	Yes No NA	Yes No NA	Yes No NA	Yes No NA	Yes No NA
Are smoking and alcohol use and habits documented?	Yes No NA	Yes No NA	Yes No NA	Yes No NA	Yes No NA	Yes No NA
Are specialists being used appropriately?	Yes No NA	Yes No NA	Yes No NA	Yes No NA	Yes No NA	Yes No NA
Are studies and labs ordered and filed correctly?	Yes No NA	Yes No NA	Yes No NA	Yes No NA	Yes No NA	Yes No NA
Are the findings consistent with the diagnoses?	Yes No NA	Yes No NA	Yes No NA	Yes No NA	Yes No NA	Yes No NA
Are the treatment plans and action consistent with diagnosis?	Yes No NA	Yes No NA	Yes No NA	Yes No NA	Yes No NA	Yes No NA
Do consultant summaries, lab results, and imaging results have the primary care physician (PCP) review?	Yes No NA	Yes No NA	Yes No NA	Yes No NA	Yes No NA	Yes No NA
Does each visit have progress notes with vital signs?	Yes No NA	Yes No NA	Yes No NA	Yes No NA	Yes No NA	Yes No NA
Is the level of care appropriate to the medical need in each visit?	Yes No NA	Yes No NA	Yes No NA	Yes No NA	Yes No NA	Yes No NA
Is the patient's name on all the pages?	Yes No NA	Yes No NA	Yes No NA	Yes No NA	Yes No NA	Yes No NA
Is there a completed immunization record?	Yes No NA	Yes No NA	Yes No NA	Yes No NA	Yes No NA	Yes No NA
Is there a current medical history and physical exam in the record?	Yes No NA	Yes No NA	Yes No NA	Yes No NA	Yes No NA	Yes No NA
Is there a follow-up plan or date for return visit for each encounter?	Yes No NA	Yes No NA	Yes No NA	Yes No NA	Yes No NA	Yes No NA
Is there a problem list in use?	Yes No NA	Yes No NA	Yes No NA	Yes No NA	Yes No NA	Yes No NA
Is there evidence of coordination of care between PCP and specialists?	Yes No NA	Yes No NA	Yes No NA	Yes No NA	Yes No NA	Yes No NA
Are there personal data?	Yes No NA	Yes No NA	Yes No NA	Yes No NA	Yes No NA	Yes No NA
Is there evidence of patient education and/or counseling for:						
Heart disease risk factors (smoking, exercise)?	N NA A1 A2 A3 A4 A5	N NA A1 A2 A3 A4 A5	N NA A1 A2 A3 A4 A5	N NA A1 A2 A3 A4 A5	N NA A1 A2 A3 A4 A5	N NA A1 A2 A3 A4 A5
Prevention of motor vehicle injury (seat belt use)?	Yes No NA	Yes No NA	Yes No NA	Yes No NA	Yes No NA	Yes No NA
Sexually transmitted disease prevention and screening (partners)?	Yes No NA	Yes No NA	Yes No NA	Yes No NA	Yes No NA	Yes No NA
HIV prevention and screening (partners)?	Yes No NA	Yes No NA	Yes No NA	Yes No NA	Yes No NA	Yes No NA
Alcoholism prevention and screening (drinks per day/week)?	Yes No NA	Yes No NA	Yes No NA	Yes No NA	Yes No NA	Yes No NA
Drug abuse prevention and screening (prescription or non)?	Yes No NA	Yes No NA	Yes No NA	Yes No NA	Yes No NA	Yes No NA

Created: [Date]

[electronic file name and path]

Medication Control

Medication	Brand Name	Price

Date Ordered	Product Name	Quantity	Price Per Unit
			$
			$
			$
			$
			$
			$
			$
			$
			$
			$
			$
			$
			$

Employee List

Name	Title	Social Security Number	Date of Hire

Quality Assurance

Check if Completed	Quality Assurance (QA) Measure	Responsible Party	Notes
☐	QA checklist with monthly evaluation	_____	_____
☐	Three levels of quality control each day patient tests are run	_____	_____
☐	Instrument calibration every 6 months or with each new lot of reagent	_____	_____
☐	Routine maintenance. Performed and documented as needed	_____	_____
☐	Consultation/interpretation of results as needed (documented)	_____	_____
☐	Generation of test report with tech signature	_____	_____
☐	Correction of errors/follow up of complaints	_____	_____
☐	Maintain QA records for 2 years	_____	_____
☐	Maintain all laboratory records at least 2 years; keep all instrument setup records forever	_____	_____
☐	Remedial action policies and procedures	_____	_____

OSHA Standards for Bloodborne Pathogens

☐	Exposure control plan	_____	_____
☐	Universal precautions for all	_____	_____
☐	Offer immunization for hepatitis B	_____	_____
☐	Sharps containers, work practice controls, hand washing	_____	_____
☐	Postexposure evaluation and follow up— retain records	_____	_____
☐	Appropriate warning labels, training	_____	_____

Miscellaneous

☐	Posted critical values and linearity readings	_____	_____
☐	Lab director's signature on all manuals	_____	_____

Check if Completed	Quality Assurance (QA) Measure	Responsible Party	Notes
	Miscellaneous (continued)		
☐	Lab director's specified personnel duties/ responsibilities	_____	_____
☐	Post licenses (personnel and laboratory)	_____	_____
☐	Normal values	_____	_____
☐	Safety manual or section in procedure manual	_____	_____
☐	Protective clothing, gloves, masks, eye protection, face shields	_____	_____
☐	Fire extinguisher charged and inspected on annual basis, employees trained	_____	_____
☐	Fire blanket	_____	_____
☐	Lids on centrifuges	_____	_____
☐	MSDS book	_____	_____
☐	Sink	_____	_____
☐	Written fire control plan and posted emergency escape route	_____	_____
☐	No smoking signs posted around flammable liquids	_____	_____
☐	Written plan of action for emergencies	_____	_____
☐	Exclusive use of refrigerators for chemicals and blood storage	_____	_____

Staff Productivity Expectations

Explanation of benefits (EOB) denial rates	%
Collection of copayments at time of service	%
Scheduling of following appointment at checkout	%
Charge entered within 24 hours	%
Collection of past-due balances	%
Registration accuracy	%
Coding accuracy	%

[electronic file name and path]

CONTROLLED DRUG DISTRIBUTION

Date	Drug Dispensed	Quantity Dispensed	Patient's Name	Initials of Person Dispensing

Controlled Drug Count for [insert name of drug]

Date	Per Count	Per Control	Difference	Count By	Difference Disposition

New Patient Census
Monthly and YTD Census of New Patients and Patients Transferred Out of the Practice

Month	Number of New Patients		Number of Patients Exiting This Month*						
	This Month	YTD	A	B	C	D	E	Total	YTD
January									
February									
March									
April									
May									
June									
July									
August									
September									
October									
November									
December									
TOTAL									

*Key: A = HMO/PPO; B = Moving; C = Referred out;
D = Other; E = Dissatisfied

chapter 4

Revenue Cycle

The revenue cycle of any medical practice begins with the physician understanding the basic financial aspects of the business. The revenue cycle involves establishing a fee schedule, determining (on the basis of community characteristics) the types of payment that will be accepted (eg, private pay, insurance, and Medicare), and deciding a percentage of the fees that will be discounted to attract a volume of business, such as that represented by a certain insurance plan.

Physicians should establish their own fee schedules on the basis of the value of the services provided rather than setting fees according to Medicare or other payment schedules. When a physician or a practice has established a fee schedule, third-party payers can be approached about negotiating the portion of fees they will pay.

To insurance carriers, patients are covered lives or insureds. The goal of insurance carriers is to pay the lowest amount possible for medical care of the insureds. The financial goal of the practice, on the other hand, is to receive the highest payment for the services provided.

Another important part of the revenue cycle is collecting the established or agreed-on fees from patient and insurance carriers with the least amount of effort. The patient portion of the bill is based on the copayment and deductible. The person at the front desk should be knowledgeable about insurance and billing issues. When possible, copayments should be collected before the patient is seen, to reduce the amount of effort necessary once their visit is completed and to eliminate any additional work on the account.

Dealing with denials of claims and appeals takes time and money from the practice. A large percentage of denials are due to incorrect information on the claim form. Claim submission and receipt of payment can be expedited by consistent implementation of clear payment policies and use of methods to acquire accurate demographic information. An electronic billing system consistent with the needs of the practice and trained reimbursement personnel are needed for accurate coding and processing claims and for receiving and recording payments.

This forms, checklists, and templates in this chapter are designed to help physicians manage the revenue cycle for the practice.

Tools for Revenue Cycle

Number	Title	Purpose	Notes
04001	Form for a Collection Activity Summary	To track collection activity for individual patients	For use by the collection personnel to track their collection activity.
04002	Form for Deposit Transactions	To record deposits	This form can be used to log deposits made with cash, check, or charge card. The aggregate data from the form can be used to compare with billing amounts and for audit and control purposes.
04003	Form for Expense Division	To calculate the allocation of expenses per physician	This form can be used to allocate practice expenses for the property, business expenses, supplies, and compensation for physicians and other staff.
04004	Form for Authorizing Write-offs	To authorize write-offs	The physician should be presented with this form along with the patient chart for review prior to approving any accounts that are to be written off.
04005	Form for Insurance Plan Data	To record data from a specific insurance plan	This form can be used to identify the insurance coverage provided in various common plans to be used as a reference by office staff.
04006	Form for a Medicare Advanced Beneficiary Notice	To notify a patient that Medicare is likely to deny payment for a service and possible reasons for the denial	This form provides a written, signed record that the patient was informed that Medicare may deny payment and the patient's agreement to pay for the service. The provider should insert the denial code number in the final column of the table.
04007	Form for a Monthly Business Summary	To monitor monthly and annual income	Data can be used to track month-to-month variations, and when data for all 12 months are recorded, they can be used to assess the year as a whole and to compare with data from previous years and practice goals.
04008	Form for a Statistical Report: Patient Accounts by Payer— Monthly	To track visits, charges, and collections according to payer, monthly	Data on this form can be used to identify and compare sources of income and the relationship of collections to charges according to payers. Data for several months or years can be used to identify trends.

Number	Title	Purpose	Notes
04009	Form for a Statistical Report: Patient Accounts by Payer—YTD	To track visits, charges, and collections according to payer, year to date	This form is to be completed by using monthly data (see Tool 04008).
04010	Form for a Statistical Report: Patient Accounts Aged AR	To track aged accounts receivable	This form can be used to break down payments according to payers and age of accounts receivable.
04011	Form for Patient Authorization—Insurance Benefits	To obtain patient authorization for the practice to apply for insurance benefits and be paid directly by the payer	For patients to release insurance benefits to a nonparticipating physician.
04012	Form for Payment Options Upon Patient Discharge	To provide staff instructions for handling payment options after a visit	This is an explanation of how employees should handle payment options.
04013	Form for Petty Cash Log	To track petty cash use	This form is used to log petty cash expenditures and calculate the balance. It also would accompany the check request to reimburse the petty cash account.
04014	Form for Petty Cash Receipt	To record petty cash expenditures	To be completed by the person in control of the petty cash fund.
04015	Form for Returned Check Tickler	To list returned checks and identify the action taken	To be completed by person who handles payments.
04016	Template for a Letter Regarding Returned Checks	To inform a patient about a returned check and the options for payment	To be completed by the person who handles payments.

Collection Activity Summary

Patient Name: _____   **ID No.:** _____

                Last   First   M

Date	Outstanding Balance	Collection Activity

Collection(s) Letter Sent

Letter 1   Date: _____

Letter 2   Date: _____

Letter 3   Date: _____

Disposition

☐   Unable to collect—Date (last attempt to collect): _____

☐   Send to collection agency—Date (sent): _____

☐   Legal action

☐   Write off

Approved By

_____   _____

              Medical Director   Date

_____   _____

              Office Manager   Date

Deposit Transactions

Date: _____

N/P*	Patient/Source	Amount	Cash	Check	Charge

*Key: N = Nonpatient receipt; P = Patient receipt

Expense Division

Key:
NA = Not applicable
S = Shared
C = Divide by collections

P = Divide by production/charges
E = Divide by employee share formula
D = Divide by physician or department

Monthly Fixed Expenses	
Divided	
	Accounting
	Office bookkeeping
	Patient billing
	Payroll service
	Automobile
	Auto lease
	Insurance
	Fuel
	Maintenance
	Building
	Exterior upkeep
	Office cleaning
	Charitable contributions
	Equipment
	Clinical equipment
	Computer
	Copier
	Purchase
	Ink
	Paper
	Repair/maintenance
	Postage meter
	Printer
	Telephone
	Insurance
	Major medical
	Individual
	Management consultants
	Initial
	Ongoing
	Marketing
	Practice promotion
	Thank-you gifts
	Yellow pages
	Parking
	Doctors
	Staff
	Pension/profit-sharing contribution
	Doctors
	Staff
	Rent
	Building
	Equipment
	Subscriptions
	Professional
	Reception area

Monthly Fixed Expenses (continued)	
Divided	
	Taxes
	City business tax
	City personal property tax
	County business tax
	County property tax
	Federal income tax
	State franchise tax
	State income tax
	Temporary Help
	Physician
	Staff
	Answering service

Fixed Expenses Occurring Regularly but Not Monthly	
Divided	
	Accountant
	Tax preparation (business)
	Tax preparation (personal)
	Conventions
	State—registration fees
	State—hotel and travel
	National—registration fees
	National—hotel and travel
	Regional—registration fees
	Dues
	National, state, and local
	Other
	Insurance (overhead)
	Professional property (comprehensive)
	Fire
	Liability
	Theft/damage
	Professional liability
	Disability—physician
	Workers' compensation
	Life/disability insurance
	Practice preservation
	Licenses
	Clinical
	City, state, and local
	Marketing
	Quarterly communications
	Newsletters

Key:

NA = Not applicable	P = Divide by production/charges
S = Shared	E = Divide by employee share formula
C = Divide by collections	D = Divide by physician or department

Expenses That Can Increase With Production	
Divided	
	Collection expenses
	Small claims court
	Clinical supplies
	Back office/clinical (eg., soap, solution, medications)
	Table paper
	Toilet paper and tissues
	Dictation
	Lab fees
	Office supplies
	Stationery
	Practice brochure
	Miscellaneous supplies and charts
	Salaries
	Physicians (draw)
	Staff
	Shared staff
	Taxes—payroll
	Uniforms
	Utilities
	Postage
	Telephone

Irregular or Unpredictable Expenses	
Divided	
	Automobile
	Continuing education
	Clinical
	Physician (spouse)
	Managerial
	Staff (clinical)
	Staff (managerial)
	Equipment Repair
	Hiring
	Advertising
	Agency fees
	Outside professional services
	Other
	Signage
	Petty cash/change

Other Expenses	
Divided	

Write-off Authorization

Patient's Name	Account Number	Total Amount Due

Date(s) of Service	Service (CPT Code)	Charge	Amount Owed

Describe collection activity: _____

_____

_____

_____

_____

Approved for collection agency: ☐ Yes ☐ No

_____   _____
Office Manager's Signature   Date

_____   _____
Managing Physician's Signature   Date

Insurance Plan Data Sheet

Insurer's Name: _____

Plan Name: _____

HMO, PPO, EPO, or Indemnity: _____

Billing Address: _____

_____

Claims Inquiry Telephone No.: _____

Provider Relations Telephone No.: _____

Medical Director Telephone No.: _____

Copayment

Office Visit: _____   Amount: _____

Well Care, Age Birth To: _____   Amount: _____

Well Care, Age To: _____

Lab Covered in Office: _____

Deductible

☐ No   ☐ Yes   Amount: _____

Required Facilities and Preauthorization Telephone Numbers

Hospital: _____

Imaging: _____

Laboratories: _____

Known Excluded Services: _____

Referral Instructions

Routine Preauthorization: _____

Hand Deliver to Specialist: _____

Services or Amount
Needing Preauthorization: _____

_____

Preauthorization No. 1
Telephone Person: _____   Telephone No.: _____

Reimbursement Rates

Medicine: _____

Lab: _____

Surgery: _____

Medicare Advanced Beneficiary Notice

Patient Name: _____   **Date of Birth:** _____

Medicare Number: _____   **Provider:** _____

Medicare will only pay for services that it determines to be "Reasonable and Necessary" under Section 1862 (a)(1) of the Medicare law. If Medicare determines that a particular service, although it would otherwise be covered, is "not reasonable and necessary" under Medicare program standards, Medicare will deny payment for that service. I believe that, in your case, Medicare is likely to deny payment. Please see the listed procedure(s) and possible reason(s) for denial of payment.

Procedure Code	Description	Date of Service	Charge	Expected Reason for Denial*

*Denial Codes Explained

Medicare usually does not pay:
1. For this service
2. For this many visits or treatments
3. For this many services within this period
4. For more than one visit a day
5. For such an extensive procedure
6. For more than one nursing home visit per month
7. For this equipment
8. For like services by more than one doctor during the same period
9. For like services by more than one doctor of the same specialty
10. Because Medicare believes and has stated that this procedure is not reasonable or necessary under recent guidelines

PATIENT AGREEMENT

My physician has notified me that, in my care, Medicare is likely to deny payment for the services identified above for the reason(s) stated. If Medicare denies payment, I agree to be personally and fully responsible for payment.

_____   _____
Signature of Patient   Date of Service

Monthly Business Summary for [insert year]

Month	No. of Days Worked	Charges	Collections	Adjust.	Accounts Receivable	Total New Patients	Total Visits	Average Visits/Day	Hospital Patients	Hospital Charges	Notes
January											
February											
March											
April											
May											
June											
July											
August											
September											
October											
November											
December											

Created: [Date]

[electronic file name and path]

Monthly Patient Account Statistical Report by Payer

Payer Class	No. of Visits	% of Total	Charges	% of Total	Collections	% of Total
BlueCross BlueShield						
Medicare						
Medical Assistance						
Medicare/Medicaid						
Medicare/BS						
Workers' Compensation						
HMO						
UHC						
Cigna						
Commercial others						
Other						
TOTAL						

Note: Break this report down by the payers specific to the office and to the level of detail most helpful for analysis.

Annual Patient Accounts Statistical Report (by Payer)
Charges and Collections by Payer Class
YTD Statistical Report

Payer Class	No. of Visits	% of Total	Charges	% of Total	Collections	% of Total
BlueCross BlueShield						
Medicare						
Medical Assistance						
Medicare/Medicaid						
Medicare/BS						
Workers' Compensation						
HMO						
UHC						
Cigna						
Commercial others						
Other						
TOTAL						

Copyright ©2009 American Medical Association

Patient Accounts Statistical Report (Aged)
Aged Accounts Receivable
Monthly Accounts Receivable Aging Report

Payer Class	Current Amt. %	30-60 Days Amt. %	61-90 Days Amt. %	91-120 Days Amt. %	120+ Days Amt. %	Total
BlueCross BlueShield						
Medicare						
Medical Assistance						
Medicare/Medicaid						
Medicare/BS						
Workers' Compensation						
HMO						
UHC						
Cigna						
Commercial others						
Other						
TOTAL						

Notes

Percentages are calculated using the total accounts receivable as the denominator.

Average Daily Charge = Total Charges ÷ Days.

Number of Days of Revenue in Receivables = Total A/R ÷ Average Daily Charge.

The total charges must have been made during the same time span specified in total days.

Patient Authorization for Release of Insurance Benefits

I, _____, hereby authorize [insert practice name] to apply for benefits

             (patient's name)

from _____ and that these benefits be made payable directly to [insert practice name]

        (insurance co. name)

(or in case of Medicare Part B benefits, to myself or to the party who accepts assignments).

I certify that the information I have reported with regard to my insurance is correct and further authorize the release
of any necessary information, including medical information for this or any related claim, to the above billing agent
(or in the case of Medicare Part B benefits, to the Social Security Administration and Centers for Medicare &
Medicaid Services and/or _____ in order to determine benefits to which

                        (other insurance company name)

I may be entitled. I permit a copy of this authorization to be used in place of the original. This authorization may be
revoked by me or the above carrier at any time in writing.

_____   _____

                 Signature   Date

Authorization to Pay Benefits to Physician

I hereby authorize payment directly to [insert practice name] of the surgical and/or medical benefits, if any,
otherwise payable to me for services described by the Attending Physician's Statement and Billing. It is understood
that any monies received from the insurance company named above, over and above my indebtedness, will be
refunded to me when my bill is paid in full. *I understand that I am financially responsible for all charges not covered
by this authorization.* I also understand should this matter be placed in the hands of an attorney for collection, I am
financially responsible for additional charges (attorney fees and court costs). I agree to pay interest on the
outstanding balance at the rate of 1.5% per month as well as reasonable attorney fees (not to exceed 20%) and
court costs with regard to the same.

_____   _____

           Signature of Policyholder   Date

Payment Options Upon Patient Discharge

Payment Method	Procedure
Cash	No identification is necessary.
Check	1. Make a copy of driver's license. 2. Staple copies to insurance/accounting copies.
Charge Card	1. Make a copy of driver's license. 2. Use electronic swipe system, and record approval number. 3. Staple copy to insurance/accounting copies.
Insurance	1. Make copy of insurance card, front and back. 2. Make a copy of driver's license. 3. Staple copies to insurance/accounting copies.
Industrial With Authorization Slip	No identification is necessary.
Industrial Without Authorization Slip (no verbal authorization obtained)	1. Make copy of insurance card, front and back. 2. Make copy of driver's license. 3. Staple copies to insurance/accounting copies.
Industrial Revisit	No identification is necessary.
Industrial Receivable (when approved)	1. Make a copy of driver's license. 2. Staple copies to insurance/accounting copies.
Partial Payment (when approved)	Follow procedures above depending on payment method. 1. Mark patient account with amount paid. 2. Note the balance due next to paid amount. 3. Make a copy of driver's license. 4. Staple copies to insurance/accounting copies. 5. Give patient a receipt showing balance due.

Petty Cash Log

Office Name: _____   Site Number: _____

| Items Purchased | Beginning Balance: | |
	Cost (of item purchased)	**Balance Total** (after subtraction of item purchased)
1.		
2.		
3.		
4.		
5.		
6.		
7.		
8.		
9.		
10.		
11.		
12.		
13.		
14.		
15.		

Instructions

- Fill in the total amount of Petty Cash for your office in Beginning Balance field.
- Subtract each item purchased, and attach receipt to log.
- When Petty Cash is depleted by 50%, attach a completed check request form and send to Accounts Payable (for Mail Log Form).

Petty Cash Receipt

Date: _____ No. _____ Check No. _____

(for replenishment)

Item Description or Service Purchased	Amount
_____	$
_____	$
_____	$
_____	$
_____	$
TOTAL	$

Charge to Account No. _____

Approved by: _____ Received by: _____

[electronic file name and path]

Returned Check Tickler

			Date:
Patient's Number	**Name**	**Action/Problem**	**Disposition**
			R D N C
			R D N C
			R D N C
			R D N C
			R D N C
			R D N C
			R D N C
			R D N C
			R D N C
			R D N C

Key: R = Received (payment satisfied); D = Done; N = Next tickler date; C = Collection

[Office Letterhead]

[Date]

Dear [Patient's name]:

This is to advise you that your check (number [insert number] for $[insert dollar amount]) has been returned twice for insufficient funds. We request that you make payment as soon as possible. The office will accept payment by cash, certified check, or credit card for your original balance of $[insert dollar amount] until [insert date]. Thereafter, we may refer the account to a collection agency plus an additional fee of $25.

Your cooperation in helping to clear up this matter is appreciated. We hope to continue to provide you with timely medical care and that you will provide us, in turn, with timely payments.

Thank you.

Sincerely,

[Office Manager]

For credit card payment, please complete the following and return to the office.

Please make payment of $_____ on my account using this credit card:

❑ Visa   ❑ MasterCard   ❑ Discover

Credit card number: _____   Expiration date: _____/_____
(month/year)

Signature: _____
(required)

Name on account: _____
(please print)

chapter 5

OSHA

Since 1992, every medical practice has been required to have an Occu-pational Safety and Health Administration (OSHA) exposure control plan. In addition, most states have additional, more stringent, require-ments for occupational safety. Adherence to OSHA regulations is as important a part of a good business as a patient medical record. Failing to meet OSHA requirements can subject a medical practice to fines of thousands of dollars per infraction. The requirements to meet the OSHA standard are available at http://www.osha.gov/pls/oshaweb/owadisp. show_document?p_table=STANDARDS&p_id=10051#.

In addition to having an OSHA exposure control plan, OSHA requires education of all employees about the plan and steps to avoid exposure to bloodborne pathogens. The training must be done within 30 days of employment and annually thereafter.

OSHA also requires the employer to offer and pay for all employees to receive hepatitis B vaccine. If an employee declines the offer, documenta-tion must be obtained.

This chapter includes forms, checklists, and templates to assist medical practices to meet the OSHA standards.

Tools for OSHA

Number	Title	Purpose	Notes
05001	Form for the Acknowledgment of Receipt of Training	To document employee education related to the OSHA exposure control plan	Retain this form in the employees personnel file as a signed acknowledgment that the employee has been trained in the listed areas.
05002	Form for an Annual OSHA Safety Walk-through of Facility	To provide a list of items to check in a safety walk-through in relation to OSHA safety standards	Use of this form provides documentation of annual compliance to the OSHA safety standards.
05003	Template for an Authorization Letter for the Release of Employee Medical Record Information to a Designated Representative	To document the employee's release of specific medical information about the injured workers medical condition as it pertains to an exposure incident.	This form identifies the specific information to be released and the purpose for which the information may be used. It also in-cludes space for the employee to restrict the authorization (eg, to a certain period).

Number	Title	Purpose	Notes
05004	Form for HIV Blood Test Consent	To inform a patient or employee after exposure about HIV and the need for a test because of accidental needle-stick or other exposure to biohazardous waste.	This form is to be read and signed by the patient or employee giving consent for an HIV test.
05005	Form for Employee Citation for Noncompliance	To document noncompliance with the OSHA Bloodborne Pathogen Standard by an employee	The explanation of the incident on this form can be used to help determine whether a change in procedures or physical characteristics of the office (eg, location of sharps containers) is needed to prevent similar incidents.
05006	Forms for an Employee Exposed to a Bloodborne Pathogen	To document exposure of an employee to a bloodborne pathogen	In addition to documenting the exposure, these forms provide for the consent of the employee and patient for blood samples to be drawn and tested for hepatitis A and B and HIV and for documenting review of the test results by a health care professional and communication of this information to the exposed employee.
05007	Form for an Employee Postexposure Incident Medical Referral Report	To record an employee's medical referral after exposure	This is a form to be filled out postexposure by the OSHA duty officer in the office.
05008	Form for Employer Referral to Employee's Health Care Provider	To document referral to an employee's health care provider after exposure to bloodborne pathogens	This checklist can help ensure that complete documentation is included when referring an employee after exposure to bloodborne pathogens.
05009	Form for an Evaluation of Exposure Incident	To evaluate an exposure incident	The data recorded on this form can be used to help prevent future incidents.
05010	Template for an Exposure Incident Reporting and Evaluation Protocol	To describe the protocol for reporting and evaluating an exposure	The protocol should be provided to employees during training so they know when and to whom an exposure incident must be reported.
05011	Template for a Hazardous Communication Labeling System	To inform employees of the meanings of labels for hazardous substances	Employers under the OSHA rules are required to notify employees of all substances used in the work place and the potential hazards associated with their use.

Number	Title	Purpose	Notes
05012	Form for Hepatitis B Vaccine Consent	To document employee consent to receive hepatitis B vaccine and to provide information about HBV infection and hepatitis B vaccine	Useful information about the Hepatitis B vaccine for the employee to read prior to agreeing or declining the vaccine.
05013	Template for a Laundry Facility Letter and Response Form	To document the laundry facility's knowledge of the presence of blood-borne pathogens and its proper handling of the laundry	A copy of this letter needs to be maintained along with your laundry service contract.
05014	Template for a Postexposure Referral Letter to a Health Care Professional	To initiate referral of an employee for evaluation and treatment after exposure to bloodborne pathogens	This letter identifies the requirements for the health care professional to whom an employee is referred.
05015	Forms for an Employee Who Refuses Hepatitis B Vaccine	To document an employee's decision to not receive hepatitis B vaccine; to document an employee's decision to continue working and risking HBV exposure after unsuccessful vaccination	Two of these forms can be used when an employee refuses hepatitis B vaccine, one of which is designed for employees who have already received the vaccine. The third form is used for employees who have received the vaccine but have not developed immunity.
05016	Checklist for OSHA Fire and Safety Training	To provide a list of items to be included in fire and safety training	An employer is required to provide this training for all employees annually.
05017	Form for Part-Time, Temporary, and Per-Diem Employee Compliance	To document that part-time, temporary, and per-diem employees understand and agree to comply with OSHA standards related to bloodborne pathogens	This form needs to be maintained as part of the employees personnel record.
05018	Form for the Employee Acknowledgment of the Exposure Control Plan	To document employee receipt of the exposure control plan	This form needs to be maintained as part of the employees personnel record.
05019	Form for a Copy of Exposure Control Plan	To be used by employees to request a hard copy of the exposure control plan	This form is also used by the employer to acknowledge receipt of the request and by the employee to acknowledge receipt of a copy of the plan.

Number	Title	Purpose	Notes
05020	Form for a Tuberculosis Protection Policy	To document the need for or lack of a need for a tuberculosis protection policy, the contents of such a policy, and the person responsible for administration of the policy, if applicable.	This policy is to be read and signed by the practice administrator, who would initial the appropriate paragraph about whether a tuberculosis protection policy is needed and would name the program administrator if a tuberculosis protection policy is needed.

Acknowledgment of Receipt of Training
OSHA 29 CFR Part 1910.1030 Occupational Exposure to Bloodborne Pathogens

Date of Training: _____   Facilitator: _____

Purpose
☐ Initial training   ☐ Orientation   ☐ Annual training   ☐ Other/retraining

Summary of Training
Training components include (but are not limited to) the following items. The employee initials each completed training component.

_____   Copy of OSHA Standard 29 CFR Part 1910.1030

_____   Explanation of the epidemiology and symptoms of bloodborne diseases

_____   Modes of transmission of bloodborne diseases

_____   Review of Exposure Control Plan

_____   Methods for recognizing tasks and other activities that may involve exposure to blood and other potentially infectious materials

_____   Use and limitations of methods that will prevent exposure

_____   Types, proper use, location, removal, handling, decontamination, and disposal of personal protective equipment

_____   Selection of personal protective equipment

_____   Benefits of being vaccinated for Hepatitis B and that the vaccine will be offered free of charge

_____   Actions to take and person to contact in an emergency involving blood or other potentially infectious materials

_____   Procedures to follow if an exposure incident occurs

_____   Postexposure evaluation and follow-up

_____   Explanation of the signs and labels required

_____   Question and answer session.

_____   Other

I have received training in the topics listed above. I was provided an opportunity to ask questions and receive answers and know that I may contact the facilitator listed above if I have additional questions.

_____   _____
Employee Name (please print)   Date

_____
Employee Signature

Annual OSHA Safety Walk-through of Facility

Facility Address: _____

In each office space, review the following areas for compliance and safety. Check Yes or No for each question, and provide a repair date, as needed, in the space provided. It is not necessary to fill out a separate page for each space, but note any deficiencies and subsequently resolve them.

Electrical Safety

Are outlets overloaded with too many plugs?	☐ Yes	☐ No	____/____/____
Are there any outlets or switches that do not work?	☐ Yes	☐ No	____/____/____
Have any 3-prong plugs been used in a 2-prong outlet?	☐ Yes	☐ No	____/____/____
Do the outlets near water sources have ground fault circuits?	☐ Yes	☐ No	____/____/____
Are there any frayed cords?	☐ Yes	☐ No	____/____/____
Are there any trip hazards related to cords?	☐ Yes	☐ No	____/____/____
Are all electrical panels accessible?	☐ Yes	☐ No	____/____/____

Falls and Slips

Are there objects in walkways?	☐ Yes	☐ No	____/____/____
Are there step stools or stepladders available for use?	☐ Yes	☐ No	____/____/____
Are there any carpeting defects?	☐ Yes	☐ No	____/____/____
Are there any loose carpets or floor mats?	☐ Yes	☐ No	____/____/____
Is there adequate lighting, especially in stairwells?	☐ Yes	☐ No	____/____/____
Are there handrails and stair treads in stairways (with more than four stairs)?	☐ Yes	☐ No	____/____/____
Are there adequate snow- and ice-removal procedures?	☐ Yes	☐ No	____/____/____

Hazard Communication

Are all secondary containers labeled correctly?	☐ Yes	☐ No	____/____/____
Are all MSDS up-to-date?	☐ Yes	☐ No	____/____/____
Do all employees know where the MSDS inventory is kept?	☐ Yes	☐ No	____/____/____
Is there a spill kit?	☐ Yes	☐ No	____/____/____

Do all employees know where the spill kit is kept? ☐ Yes ☐ No _____/_____/_____

Are all exits labeled correctly? (Exit and Not an Exit) ☐ Yes ☐ No _____/_____/_____

Are oxygen and other compressed gas cylinders maintained? ☐ Yes ☐ No _____/_____/_____

Are oxygen and other compressed gas cylinders secured in a safe condition? ☐ Yes ☐ No _____/_____/_____

Are there mounted eyewash stations within 25 feet or 15 seconds of any toxic or corrosive materials? ☐ Yes ☐ No _____/_____/_____

Are the eyewash stations flushed for a minimum of 1 minute weekly? ☐ Yes ☐ No _____/_____/_____

Is the temperature of the water for the eyewash station 100°F or less? ☐ Yes ☐ No _____/_____/_____

Is the OSHA 300 Form completed and accessible? (If not exempt) ☐ Yes ☐ No _____/_____/_____

Was the OSHA 300-A Form posted February through March? (If not exempt) ☐ Yes ☐ No _____/_____/_____

Is a first-aid kit available? ☐ Yes ☐ No _____/_____/_____

Are chemicals, medicines, specimens, and supplies stored separately from food? ☐ Yes ☐ No _____/_____/_____

Is the hazardous materials refrigerator labeled: "NO FOOD OR BEVERAGE ALLOWED"? ☐ Yes ☐ No _____/_____/_____

Fire Safety

Are there fire extinguishers? (5 lb, ABC rating) ☐ Yes ☐ No _____/_____/_____

Have they been serviced annually? ☐ Yes ☐ No _____/_____/_____

Does the practice have a policy for immediate evacuation of the building in the event of a fire? ☐ Yes ☐ No _____/_____/_____

If yes, no fire drills are required.

If no, have fire drills been performed? ☐ Yes ☐ No _____/_____/_____

Emergency Plan

Does the practice have an emergency action plan? ☐ Yes ☐ No _____/_____/_____

Is it in writing? (fewer than 10 employees requires a verbal plan only) ☐ Yes ☐ No _____/_____/_____

Does the emergency plan include procedures for fire, earthquake, hurricane, and tornado? ☐ Yes ☐ No _____/_____/_____

Are exit routes posted? □ Yes □ No _____/_____/_____

Bloodborne Pathogen

Are there sharps containers? □ Yes □ No _____/_____/_____

Are the sharps containers filled past the full line? □ Yes □ No _____/_____/_____

Are all regulated waste containers covered and labeled correctly? □ Yes □ No _____/_____/_____

Are all regulated waste containers, including sharps, disposed of correctly? □ Yes □ No _____/_____/_____

Is the Bloodborne Pathogen Manual updated? □ Yes □ No _____/_____/_____

Is there adequate PPE? □ Yes □ No _____/_____/_____

Are all employees aware of proper use of PPE? □ Yes □ No _____/_____/_____

Is contaminated laundry handled properly? □ Yes □ No _____/_____/_____

Is the Needle-Stick Log completed and accessible? □ Yes □ No _____/_____/_____

Was it posted for the months of February to April? □ Yes □ No _____/_____/_____

Have all employees who have potential exposure been offered or received a hepatitis B vaccination? □ Yes □ No _____/_____/_____

　　Are there records of this? □ Yes □ No _____/_____/_____

　　Are there signed declinations, if applicable? □ Yes □ No _____/_____/_____

Other

Are all X-ray protocols being followed? □ Yes □ No _____/_____/_____

Has the safety committee met and are minutes accessible? □ Yes □ No _____/_____/_____

Release of Employee Medical Record Information

I, _____, hereby authorize _____
          (full name of worker/patient)   (individual/organization holding medical records)

to release to _____, the following medical
            (individual or organization authorized to receive the medical information)

information from my personal medical records: _____

_____
                         (describe generally the information desired to be released)

I give my permission for this medical information to be used for the following purpose:

_____

_____
                                   (describe the purpose)

but I do not give permission for any other use or redisclosure of this information.

Note: Several extra lines are provided below so that you can place additional restrictions on this authorization letter if you want to. You may leave these lines blank. On the other hand, you may want to (1) specify a particular expiration date for this letter (for example, one year); (2) describe medical information to be created in the future that you intend to be covered by this authorization letter; or (3) describe portions of the medical information in your records that you do not intend to be released as a result of this letter.

_____

_____

_____

_____

_____

_____

_____
Full Name of Employee or Legal Representative

_____   _____
Signature of Employee or Legal Representative   Date of Signature

Consent Form: Blood Test for Human Immunodeficiency Virus (HIV) Antibody Information Sheet

WHAT IS HIV?

HIV is the virus that is the probable cause of acquired immunodeficiency syndrome (AIDS).

WHAT IS THE HIV ANTIBODY TEST?

The HIV antibody test is a lab test done on a blood specimen taken from you by a physician, nurse, or technician. This is not a diagnostic test for AIDS. A positive test means that you have been infected with the virus that causes AIDS. This test usually becomes positive within 6 months of exposure.

WHAT DOES A POSITIVE TEST RESULT MEAN?

If the results of the initial test are positive, further tests will be conducted to confirm this initial result. A positive confirmatory test means that it is almost certain that you are a carrier of the AIDS virus. This means that you can transmit this virus to others by intimate sexual contact, by sharing needles, and through blood and organ donation. A pregnant woman can pass this infection on to her child. A woman who is breastfeeding may also pass this infection along to her child. A positive test result does not mean that you have AIDS or that you will develop AIDS. However, studies have shown that a large percentage of people who show positive test results will develop AIDS-related complex or AIDS within 5 to 6 years.

WHAT DOES A NEGATIVE RESULT MEAN?

A negative test result means that no antibody to HIV has been detected in your blood. This does not necessarily mean that you have not been exposed to or infected with HIV. Although you may have been infected with HIV, it is possible that your body has not yet made an antibody to the virus. Since the blood tests are not 100% accurate, it is possible that the test has failed to detect the antibody (this is known as a false-negative result).

CONSENT

I have read or someone has read to me the information on this sheet. I have been provided with information about prevention and transmission of AIDS. I have been informed about the nature of the blood tests, their purpose, their expected benefits and uses, and the possible need for additional tests and have been given the opportunity to ask questions about these tests and their results. My questions have been answered to my satisfaction. I also understand that if confirmatory tests are positive, counseling will be made available to me.

By signing below, I acknowledge that I have received all the information I need concerning the blood tests. I understand that to the extent possible, my physician will not disclose the results of these tests to others except as required by law or as necessary to safeguard the well-being of other health care professionals or employees involved in my medical care or treatment or other persons at risk. However, I do understand that the absolute confidentiality of the test results cannot be guaranteed, although all measures required by law to ensure the confidentiality of the results of the blood test will be followed. I understand the results will be placed in my medical record.

On the above basis, I consent to the performance of a blood test to detect antibodies to the human immunodeficiency virus (HIV).

_____   _____
Signature of Patient or Person Authorized to Consent   Date
for Patient and Relationship to Patient

_____   _____
Signature of Witness   Date

_____   _____
Signature of Physician/Counselor   Date

Employee Citation for Noncompliance

INSTRUCTIONS

This form should be used by the employer or authorized representative to cite employees for noncompliance incidents related to the OSHA Bloodborne Pathogens Standard and the employer's exposure control plan.

Date of Incident: _____

Employee ID: _____

Social Security Number: _____

Employee Name: _____ _____ _____

                              Last Name   First Name   Middle

EXPLANATION OF NONCOMPLIANCE INCIDENT

_____

_____

_____

_____

_____   _____

Signature of Employer or Authorized Representative   Date

TO BE COMPLETED BY EMPLOYEE

By signing below I acknowledge that this citation has been reviewed with me and the proper procedures for compliance related to this incident have been discussed with me.

_____   _____

              Employee's Signature   Date

Employee's Comments:

_____

_____

Employee Postexposure Incident Report: Confidential

Name of Employee: _____

Date and Time of Incident: _____

During the course of my treatment or contact with a patient of this practice, I was inadvertently exposed to a potentially infectious bodily fluid. The details of this incident are described below:

_____

_____

_____

_____

I have been informed of the postexposure protocol in place in this office and I plan to complete all of the required steps to ensure complete compliance with the OSHA Bloodborne Pathogen Exposure Control Plan.

NOTE: No employee is required to seek medical attention or have any clinical laboratory tests, *but* it is strongly advised that each employee who has had an exposure to bloodborne pathogens follow the recommended OSHA postexposure protocol steps. In addition, all postexposure protocol steps are at **no cost** to the employee.

Signature: _____

Source Patient Information

Name or Chart Number of Source Patient: _____

Has the patient been informed of this incident by the   ☐ Yes   ☐ No
employee or the patient's physician?

Has the patient been requested to submit to blood testing   ☐ Yes   ☐ No
for HIV, HBV, and HCV?

Consent to Perform Laboratory Testing: Patient

I have been informed that during the performance of his/her duties, an employee of this practice was exposed to my bodily fluid. In order to assess and minimize the risk to the exposed employee, I give my consent for a blood sample to be drawn by a licensed laboratory to detect the presence of an infectious organism including hepatitis B, hepatitis C, and HIV.

I have been advised of the side effects of the blood draw. I also understand that the tests will be conducted in a confidential manner to protect my identity. I also understand that this test will be at no cost to me.

Patient's Name: _____

Patient's Signature: _____

Date: _____

Witness's Name: _____

Witness's Signature: _____

Date: _____

Consent to Perform Laboratory Testing: Employee

On _____, I was inadvertently exposed to a potentially infectious bodily fluid. In order to assess
        (date)
and to minimize the risks associated with this exposure, I give my consent for blood to be drawn from me to detect the presence of disease including hepatitis B, hepatitis C, and HIV.

I have been advised of the side effects of a blood draw. I also understand that the tests will be conducted in a confidential manner by a licensed laboratory to protect my identity.

The results may be made **only** to my personal physician and/or the licensed health care professional, who will conduct the postexposure and follow-up evaluations.

Employee's Name: _____

Employee's Signature: _____

Date: _____

Witness's Name: _____

Witness's Signature: _____

Date: _____

Health Care Professional's Written Opinion: Confidential

This report must be presented to the exposed employee within 15 days from the completion of the health care professional's evaluation.

Employee's Name: _____

Date of Exposure: _____

Source Patient's Serologic Status

HBsAG	☐ Positive	☐ Negative	☐ Unknown
HCsAG	☐ Positive	☐ Negative	☐ Unknown
HIV	☐ Positive	☐ Negative	☐ Unknown

Has the employee received hepatitis B vaccine?

☐ Yes ☐ No

Is there any medical reason why the employee should not receive the hepatitis B vaccine, if he/she has not already received it?

NOTE: Only comment on the ability to receive the HBV vaccine. All other findings are to remain confidential.

☐ No
☐ Yes (if yes, explain): _____

_____

_____

I have informed the employee named above of the results of my medical evaluation. The employee is fully aware of any medical conditions that may result from the exposure to blood or other potentially infectious material. The employee understands that further medical treatment may or may not be required.

Physician's Name: _____

Physician's Signature: _____

Date: _____

Employee's Postexposure Incident Medical Referral Report: Confidential

Date _____

Employee Name _____

Job Description _____

Exposure Determination Category _____

Employee Hepatitis B Vaccine Status _____

Date Received _____ Date Refused _____

Date documentation received and filed in employee's confidential medical
record if antibody testing indicated employee is immune   _____

Date documentation received and filed in employee's confidential medical
record if the vaccine is contraindicated for medical reasons   _____

Other relevant medical information _____

_____

Description of employee's duties at the time of the exposure incident _____

_____

_____

Description of how incident occurred _____

_____

_____

Source

Source Name _____

	Source HBV Status	Source HIV Status	Source HCV Status
Indicate date positive	_____	_____	
Indicate date negative	_____	_____	
Check if unknown	☐	☐	☐
Check if pending	☐	☐	☐

Completed By

Name _____ Title _____
        (print or type)   (print or type)

Signature _____

Employer Referral to Employee's Health Care Provider

The checked terms represent supporting documents with this referral.

☐ Copy of OSHA Standard (CFR 1910.1030)

☐ Confidential exposure incident report:
—A description of the exposed employee's duties as they relate to the exposure incident
—Documentation of the route(s) of exposure and circumstances under which exposure occurred

☐ Source individual HIV/HBV/HBC status (if known)

☐ All medical records relevant to the appropriate treatment of the employee, including vaccination status

☐ Source individual identification (if known)

Evaluation of Exposure Incident
CONFIDENTIAL

1. Date of incident: _____   Date form completed: _____

2. Time of incident: _____   Time form completed: _____

3. Name of individual exposed: _____

4. Name of source of exposure: _____

5. Description of employee's duties during the exposure incident:

    _____

6. Description of how the incident occurred:

    _____

    _____

    _____

7. The specific route of exposure was

    ☐ Needle stick with contaminated needle to _____

    ☐ Piercing of skin with contaminated sharp to _____

    ☐ Splashing/spraying of blood or other potentially infectious materials to _____

    ☐ Other (describe) _____

8. Check the workplace control(s) that were examined in the investigation of this exposure incident and your comments/findings.

	Control	**Comments/Findings**
☐ Universal precautions	_____	_____
☐ Engineering controls	_____	_____
☐ Workplace controls	_____	_____
☐ Personal protective equipment	_____	_____
☐ Housekeeping	_____	_____
☐ Other (specify)	_____	_____

9. Please list any changes that may minimize future exposure for similar settings.

Specific Change	**Date Implemented**
_____	_____
_____	_____
_____	_____
_____	_____
_____	_____

10. Employee's comments

_____

_____

_____

_____   _____
Signature of Employee   Date

11. Employer's comments

_____

_____

_____

_____   _____
Signature of Employer   Date

Name and title of person completing this form: _____

Date form was completed: _____

Copy to: _____   Employee's Confidential Medical File: _____

Exposure Incident Reporting and Evaluation Protocol

1. Upon exposure to blood or other potentially infectious material, the employee will wash hands and any other skin surface that may have been exposed and will flush with water mucous membranes that may have been in contact with blood or other potentially infectious materials, as soon as feasible after exposure.

2. Following the washing and/or flushing previously described, the employee will report the exposure incident to one of the following:

   A.   [insert contact name and information]

   B.   [insert contact name and information]

3. A confidential employee's exposure incident medical report will be completed by one of the following:

   A.   [insert contact name and information]

   B.   [insert contact name and information]

4. A confidential Employee Postexposure Employer Referral to Health Care Professional Packet will be completed by one of the following:

   A.   [insert contact name and information]

   B.   [insert contact name and information]

5. A copy from the written opinion of the health care provider must be provided to the employer within 15 days of the medical evaluation.

6. One copy of the written opinion is given to the employee, and a second copy is filed with the employee medical record.

7. The exposure incident is evaluated, and a report of the incident must be completed.

Hazardous Communication Labeling System

The National Fire Protection Association (NFPA) has developed a rating system for identifying the Health, Flammability, and Reactivity hazards of a chemical. The National Paint and Coating Association has also prepared a rating system similar to the NFPA rating.

The following codes are described in detail on the Hazard Material Identification Chart.

Health: Blue

4   DANGEROUS: Can be fatal on minimal exposure. Need special protection equipment.

3   WARNING: Protect skin, do not inhale, corrosive, or toxic.

2   WARNING: Can be harmful if inhaled or absorbed.

1   CAUTION: Can be irritating.

0   Very minimal, no hazard.

Reactivity: Yellow

4   DANGEROUS: Can explode at room temperature.

3   DANGEROUS: Can explode if substance is shocked, heated in confined conditions, or mixed with water.

2   WARNING: Unstable. Substance can react if mixed with water.

1   CAUTION: Can react if heated or mixed with water.

0   STABLE: Does not react with water.

Flammability: Red

4   DANGEROUS: Extremely flammable liquid or gas.

3   WARNING: Flash point is below 100°F. Flammable.

2   CAUTION: Flash point is between 100°F and 200°F.

1   Flash point is at or higher than 200°F.

0   Normally stable. Not combustible.

Consent Form for Hepatitis B Vaccine Information Sheet

WHAT IS HEPATITIS B?

Hepatitis B is an infection of the liver caused by the hepatitis B virus (HBV). Acute hepatitis usually begins with mild symptoms such as loss of appetite, extreme tiredness, nausea, vomiting, stomach pain, dark urine, and jaundice (yellow eyes and skin). Skin rashes and joint pain may also occur.

Young adults make up the largest group of individuals who catch the infection. Between 6% and 10% of those who catch hepatitis B become chronic carriers (have the virus in their blood for more than 6 months) and may be able to infect others for a long time. About 25% of these carriers go on to develop chronic active hepatitis, which often induces cirrhosis of the liver, leading to death by liver failure. HBV carriers also have a high incidence of cancer of the liver.

WHAT IS THE HEPATITIS B VACCINE?

The vaccine can be made from HBV particles that have been purified from the blood of carriers. The process used in this method kills all types of viruses found in human blood, including the virus that causes AIDS. The vaccine can also be produced through genetic engineering from baker's yeast cells. These recombinant vaccines do not contain human blood products.

HOW IS THE HEPATITIS B VACCINE GIVEN?

The vaccine is administered by injection on three separates dates. The first two doses are usually given 1 month apart and the final dose 5 months after the second. The vaccine is 85% to 95% effective in preventing hepatitis B infection after the third dose. In normal healthy adults and children, protection lasts at least 7 years.

WHO SHOULD GET HEPATITIS B VACCINE?

It is recommended that all persons who are at high risk of catching HBV infection receive the vaccine. These groups include the following: health care and public safety workers who are exposed to blood or blood products; clients and staff of institutions for the mentally disabled; users of illicit injectable drugs; household, sexual, and other contacts of HBV carriers; adoptees and persons from areas with high rates of hepatitis B; travelers to areas with high rates of hepatitis B; and inmates of long-term correctional facilities.

WHAT IF I HAVE ALREADY BEEN EXPOSED TO HBV?

The hepatitis B vaccine series should be started at the same time as other therapy, which is primarily treatment with hepatitis B immune globulin (HBIG). It is particularly recommended for the following groups: infants born to mothers who have a positive blood test for hepatitis B surface antigen (HBsAg), persons having accidents involving HBsAg-positive blood, infants younger than 1 year whose mother or primary care giver has HBsAg-positive blood, and persons having sexual contact with someone who has HBsAg-positive blood.

ARE THERE ANY POSSIBLE RISKS DURING PREGNANCY?

No data are available about the safety of the vaccine for unborn babies; however, there should be no risk since the vaccine contains only particles that do not cause hepatitis B infection. A pregnant woman who gets hepatitis B infection transmits a chronic infection to her newborn child.

CONSENT

I have read or someone has read to me the information on this sheet about hepatitis B and hepatitis B vaccine. I have been given the opportunity to ask questions, which were answered to my satisfaction. I understand that if I get sick during the 4 weeks after receiving the vaccine, I should immediately report this fact to my physician. I believe I understand the benefits and risks of the hepatitis B vaccine and request that it be given to me.

_____   _____
Signature   Date

DATE: [insert date]

TO: [insert name of company or service representative]

FROM: [insert physician office name or contact person]

Because we ship contaminated laundry to your facility, compliance with the OSHA Bloodborne Pathogens Standard, CFR 1910.1030, requires that our employer determine whether your facility utilizes universal precautions in the handling of all laundry.

Please complete the attached form and return to our office within 15 days of the date of this letter. We must have this form on file no later than [insert date obtained from compliance calendar] to be in compliance with the OSHA standard.

Previous Hepatitis B Vaccination

I am declining the hepatitis B vaccine at this time because I have already received the series of vaccinations.

I understand that as a result of my occupational exposure to blood or other potentially infectious materials, I may be at risk of acquiring a hepatitis B virus (HBV) infection. I have been given the opportunity to be vaccinated with hepatitis B vaccine, at no charge to myself. However, I decline the hepatitis B vaccine at this time. I understand that by declining this vaccine, I continue to be at risk of acquiring Hepatitis B, a serious disease. If in the future I continue to have occupational exposure to blood or other potentially infectious materials, and I want to be vaccinated with hepatitis B vaccine, I can receive the vaccination series at no charge to me.

_____   _____
Employee's Signature   Date

_____   _____
Witness's Signature   Date

Received by the practice:

_____   _____
Signature   Date

Is there a record of this vaccination series?   ☐ Yes   ☐ No

Is there a copy on file to attach to this declination?   ☐ Yes   ☐ No

DATE: [insert date]

TO: [insert name]

FROM:[insert name]

Dear Health Care Professional/Colleague:

[Insert employee's full name] has been referred to your office because of an occupational exposure incident. Compliance with the OSHA standard CFR 1910.1030 (Bloodborne Pathogen Standard effective March 6, 1992) requires that he/she be seen by a health care professional for immediate and confidential postexposure evaluation. A copy of the standard accompanies this letter.

In compliance with the OSHA guidelines, we are asking that you provide our employee with the following:

- An evaluation of the exposure incident
- Testing for HBV/HIV of the employee and the source individual, if not already done
- Results of all testing
- Postexposure prophylaxis, when medically indicated, as recommended by the US Public Health Service
- Counseling
- An evaluation of the reported illness
- A complete health care professional written opinion and return to employer

The OSHA guidelines mandate that I receive from you the following documentation:

- A written opinion that is limited to whether hepatitis B vaccination is indicated for an employee and whether the employee has received such vaccination.
- A statement that the employee has been told about any medical condition resulting from exposure to blood or other potentially infectious materials that requires further evaluation and treatment.

Hepatitis B Vaccination Declination (Mandatory)

I understand that as a result of my occupational exposure to blood or other potentially infectious materials, I may be at risk of acquiring hepatitis B virus (HBV) infection. I have been given the opportunity to be vaccinated with hepatitis B vaccine at no charge to myself. However, I decline the hepatitis B vaccine at this time. I understand that by declining this vaccine, I continue to be at risk of acquiring hepatitis B, a serious disease. If in the future I continue to have occupational exposure to blood or other potentially infectious materials and I want to be vaccinated with hepatitis B vaccine, I can receive the vaccination series at no charge to me.

_____   _____
                Employee's Signature   Date

_____   _____
                Witness's Signature   Date

Received by the practice:

_____   _____
                   Signature   Date

Previous Hepatitis B Vaccination

I am declining the hepatitis B vaccine at this time because I have already received the series of vaccinations.

I understand that as a result of my occupational exposure to blood or other potentially infectious materials, I may be at risk of acquiring a hepatitis B virus (HBV) infection. I have been given the opportunity to be vaccinated with hepatitis B vaccine, at no charge to myself. However, I decline the hepatitis B vaccine at this time. I understand that by declining this vaccine, I continue to be at risk of acquiring Hepatitis B, a serious disease. If in the future I continue to have occupational exposure to blood or other potentially infectious materials, and I want to be vaccinated with hepatitis B vaccine, I can receive the vaccination series at no charge to me.

_____   _____
Employee's Signature   Date

_____   _____
Witness's Signature   Date

Received by the practice:

_____   _____
Signature   Date

Is there a record of this vaccination series?   ☐ Yes   ☐ No
Is there a copy on file to attach to this declination? ☐ Yes   ☐ No

Hepatitis B Virus Inoculation Waiver
(For Unsuccessful Immunizations Only)

My employer has provided the HBV vaccination to me at no cost; however, I did not develop immunity to HBV, even after repeated boosters, according to the laboratory tests performed.

It is my intention to continue to perform duties that might expose me to material infected with HBV, even though tests have indicated that I am not immune to HBV.

I agree not to hold this facility or its owners liable (other than through my rights afforded through workers' compensation coverage) if I should contract HBV while on the job.

| _____ | _____ |
| Employee's Signature | Date |

| _____ | _____ |
| Witness's Signature | Date |

Received by the practice:

| _____ | _____ |
| Signature | Date |

OSHA Fire and Safety Training

To be conducted on initial assignment.

Check if Completed		Responsible Party	Notes
☐	What to do if employee discovers a fire	_____	_____
☐	Demonstration of alarm, if more than one type exists	_____	_____
☐	How to recognize fire exits	_____	_____
☐	Evacuation routes	_____	_____
☐	Assisting employees and patients with disabilities	_____	_____
☐	Measures to contain fire (eg, closing office doors, windows in immediate vicinity)	_____	_____
☐	Head count procedures (see emergency action plan for details)	_____	_____
☐	Return to building after the "all-clear" signal	_____	_____
☐	Types of fires	_____	_____
☐	Types of fire prevention equipment	_____	_____
☐	Location of fire prevention equipment	_____	_____
☐	How to use fire prevention equipment	_____	_____
☐	Limitations of fire prevention equipment	_____	_____
☐	Proper care and maintenance of assigned fire prevention equipment	_____	_____
☐	Location of exit doors, evacuation plan, and the use of fire extinguisher	_____	_____

Part-time, Temporary, and Per-diem Employee Compliance

REQUIREMENTS

As stated in OSHA Instruction CPL 02-02-069 (Office of Health Compliance Assistance), "Part-time, temporary, and health care workers known as 'per diem' employees are covered by this standard."

INSTRUCTIONS

1. This form should be used by the employer to document that a part-time, temporary, or per-diem employee fully understands and agrees to comply with OSHA's Bloodborne Pathogens Standards.

2. This form should be retained in the employer's files for the duration of the employee's employment plus 30 years.

Date of Initial Assignment: _____

Employee Name: _____ _____ _____
                        last name   first name   middle

Social Security Number: _____

TO BE COMPLETED BY PART-TIME, TEMPORARY, AND HEALTH CARE WORKERS KNOWN AS "PER DIEM" EMPLOYEES

By signing below I confirm that:
- I have been provided training from my employer as required by the OSHA Bloodborne Pathogens Standard, CFR 1910.1030.
- I have been offered the hepatitis B vaccination.
- I have received training on this employer's exposure control plan and agree to adhere to the policies, procedures, and controls in this plan.

_____   _____
              Employee's Signature   Date

Employee Acknowledgment of Exposure Control Plan

I acknowledge receiving a copy of the Exposure Control Plan for [insert office/employer name].

I understand that I must review the plan in its entirety and comply with the plan's requirements.

_____   _____

Employee's Signature   Date

Statement of Availability—Request for Copy of Exposure Control Plan

REQUIREMENTS

As stated in OSHA instruction CPL 02-02-069 (Office of Health Compliance Assistance), the location of the exposure control plan may be adapted to the circumstances of a particular workplace provided that the employees can access a copy at the workplace, during the workshift 9:00 A.M. through 5:00 P.M. If the plan is maintained on computer, employees must be trained to operate the computer. In accordance with 29 CFR 1910.1030, a hard copy of the exposure control plan shall be made available to the employees within 15 working days of the employee's request.

INSTRUCTIONS

1. Notify each employee of the location of this plan.
2. For each employee who requests a hard copy of this plan, have the employee complete the request portion of this form.
3. The employer should acknowledge receipt of this form by signing the request portion of this form on the date received.
4. Once the hard copy of this plan is provided to the employee, have the employee sign the request portion of this form to acknowledge receipt of the plan.

REQUEST FOR COPY OF EXPOSURE CONTROL PLAN

I, _____, as an employee of this facility, request a hard copy of the exposure control plan for this facility. I understand that this exposure control plan is confidential and proprietary to this facility and agree to handle it accordingly.

_____   _____
Employee Signature   Date of Request

_____   _____
Employer Signature   Date of Receipt
for Acknowledgment of Receipt of This Request

RECEIPT OF COPY OF EXPOSURE CONTROL PLAN

I, _____, per my request for a hard copy of the exposure control plan for this office on _____, have received this copy.

_____   _____
Employee Signature   Date of Receipt

Tuberculosis Protection Policy

Practice Name: _____

Practice Address: _____

_____

_____ Because of the nature of the services provided by this practice and the demographic characteristics of the patients served, we have determined that at this time our workers are not at risk for exposure to tuberculosis (TB) and therefore a TB control plan and respiratory protection are not necessary. Should this change in the future, we will implement a TB control plan using CDC's 1994 guidelines and a respiratory protection policy in compliance with OSHA Standard 29 CFR 1910.134.

_____ We have evaluated the procedures we perform and the demographic characteristics of the patients we serve and have determined that there is the potential for undiagnosed TB patients to enter our facility. However, we cannot protect against the unknown. At this time, our policy is to immediately refer anyone with a suspected case of TB to the public health department, a pulmonologist, or an infectious disease specialist. Therefore, a TB control plan and respiratory protection are not required at this time. Should this change, we will implement a TB control plan according to CDC guidelines and a respiratory protection policy in compliance with OSHA Standard 29 CFR 1910.134.

_____ We have determined that a TB control plan and respiratory protection are not necessary in this setting. However, we will allow workers to voluntarily wear dust masks to protect themselves against potential exposure to TB, SARS, or other airborne infections, chemicals, or irritants. Employees who choose respiratory protection voluntarily must read and sign Appendix D, which follows this policy.

_____ Because of the nature of the services provided by this practice and the demographic characteristics of the patients served, we have determined that at this time our workers are at risk for exposure to TB and therefore a TB control plan and respiratory protection are necessary. Should this change in the future, we will discontinue the respiratory protection policy. As a result of this determination, we will develop and implement a policy in compliance with OSHA Standard 29 CFR 1910.134. We will appoint a staff member to administer the program and will provide that individual with the resources needed. Our policy will include all the required elements, including:

1. Evaluation of staff positions to determine which workers require protection.

2. Medical evaluation of all affected workers to determine their ability to use the respirators. Evaluations will be performed by a physician or other licensed health care provider, free of charge to the employee, and all findings will remain confidential.

3. Consistent use of appropriate NIOSH-certified respirators, provided free of charge to employees.

4. Training, also free of charge to all employees, to ensure that affected employees understand the importance and limitations of the respirators, how to properly don and check them, and when they should be replaced.

Should an employee become exposed to TB, we will notify the employee and offer the appropriate follow-up. Should a current employee or a patient be diagnosed with active TB, we will implement the policy found elsewhere in this manual.

This practice has appointed _____ as program administrator, charged with the responsibility and given the necessary authority and resources for developing and overseeing the respiratory protection program if applicable.

_____   _____
Practice Administrator   Date

chapter 6

CLIA

The Clinical Laboratory Improvement Amendments of 1988 (CLIA) require that all practices that operate a laboratory within their offices must provide standards to correctly identify, process, and handle specimens. Furthermore, CLIA also requires maintaining equipment and showing evidence of such maintenance. This chapter provides the forms, checklists, and templates that can be used to comply with CLIA.

In addition to complying with regulations about in-office laboratory facilities, it is important for the practice to ensure that laboratory charges are properly billed. One way to ascertain that all tests performed in the office are properly billed is to compare the laboratory log (Tool 06005) with encounter records and checkout reports. The comparison could be done daily or as indicated by the testing volume in the practice.

Tools for CLIA

Number	Title	Purpose	Notes
06001	Checklist for Correct Blood Collection Tubes	To describe blood collection tubes by color of the stopper and their uses	This checklist identifies the anticoagulant, if any, in the tubes; the sizes of tubes available; the minimum volume, if applicable; and the tests for which samples in the various tubes are used.
06002	Form for an Equipment Record Log	To record data, primarily about purchase, for equipment in the laboratory	This form is to be completed for each piece of equipment. The log should be stored safely; copies of receipts and warranty information might also be kept with the log.
06003	Form for Equipment Calibration Requirements	To log calibration requirements for laboratory equipment and track completion of required calibration	Each piece of equipment has its own log sheet.
06004	Form for an Equipment Repair Record	To track the repairs and repair costs for laboratory equipment	Each piece of equipment has its own repair record.
06005	Form for a Laboratory Log	To track performance of laboratory tests and review and recording of test results	A part of the laboratory quality assurance program.

Number	Title	Purpose	Notes
06006	Checklist for a CLIA New Laboratory Start-up	To assist a practice to open a laboratory	A checklist to help organize the laboratory start-up process.
06007	Checklist for the Preparation for CLIA Recertification and/ or State Clinical Laboratory Surveys	To indicate the items needed for a survey for recertification by CLIA and/or for a state clinical laboratory survey	A very helpful checklist for any laboratory.
06008	Template for Reporting Laboratory and Test Results to Patients	To document patient notification of test results	A part of the laboratory quality assurance program.

Checklist for Correct Blood Collection Tubes

☐   **RED STOPPER (or Gray and Red Stopper—SST; Note: SST = serum separation tube)**

Anticoagulant:	None
Sizes:	10 mL, 3 mL, and 0.8 mL microtainer
Minimum tube volume:	None
Primary test:	Most general and special chemistries requiring serum

DO NOT SHAKE OR INVERT THIS TUBE. Shaking will cause hemolysis of the red blood cells and can affect test results.

☐   **LAVENDER STOPPER**

Anticoagulant:	EDTA
Sizes:	5.0 mL, and microtainer 0.25 to 0.50 mL
Minimum tube volume:	1 mL in 5.0-mL tube
	Microtainer tube-between the two purple lines
Primary test:	CBC, CEA, T cell studies, ammonia (on ice) (blood/plasma)

☐   **BLUE STOPPER**

Anticoagulant:	Sodium citrate
Sizes:	4.5 mL and 2.7 mL
Minimum tube volume:	These tubes must be full
Primary test:	Coagulation tests (PT, PTT, fibrinogen)

☐   **GRAY STOPPER**

Anticoagulant:	Potassium or lithium oxalate or sodium fluoride
Sizes:	5.0 ml only
Minimum tube volume:	1.5 ml
Primary test:	Lactic acid (on ice), alcohol (blood/plasma)

☐   **GREEN STOPPER**

Anticoagulant:	Sodium lithium and ammonium heparin
Sizes:	5.0 mL and 2.7 mL
Minimum tube volume:	One-third the full volume
Primary test:	Chromosome studies (blood/plasma)

Equipment Record Log

Equipment Record Number: _____

Type of Equipment: _____

Vendor Name: _____

Vendor Address: _____

_____

_____

Telephone Number: _____

Manufacturer's Name: _____

Trade Name: _____

Date Purchased: _____ / _____ / _____   **Cost:** $ _____

Equipment Calibration Requirements

Equipment Name_____

Model Number_____

Serial Number_____

Required		Done	
Date	Other Criteria	Performed By	Date

Repair Record

Equipment Name_____

Model Number_____

Serial Number_____

Warranty Date and Parts Covered: _____

Date	Problem	Repair Performed	Cost

Laboratory Log

PATIENT		TEST	I/O	PHYSICIAN or NURSE REVIEW		RECORDED RESULT CHART	
NAME	NUMBER			DATE	BY	DATE	BY

[electronic file name and path]

Created: [Date]

CLIA New Laboratory Start-up

Check if Completed		Responsible Party	Notes
☐	Apply for licensure of laboratory (have copies available in CLIA manual)	_____	_____
☐	Apply for licensure for personnel (have copies available in CLIA manual)	_____	_____
☐	BBR replies, send readiness letter	_____	_____
☐	Set-up inspection	_____	_____

Set-up of Instruments

☐	Linearity for each analyte—post reportable range	_____	_____
☐	Ten of same pt. run for precision— Calculate mean, coefficient of variation (CV), standard deviation (SD)	_____	_____
☐	Three levels of QC run 10× each— Calculate mean, CV, SD	_____	_____
☐	10 Split samples run with reference instrument or laboratory—Compare results	_____	_____

Personnel Records

☐	Resume or credentials	_____	_____
☐	License copy or proof of application	_____	_____
☐	HBsAg immunization records or signed waiver	_____	_____
☐	Monitors for employee competence— evaluations	_____	_____

Procedure Manual

☐	Specimen collection/rejection criteria	_____	_____
☐	Package inserts for reagents and quality control material	_____	_____
☐	Critical value action procedures	_____	_____
☐	Normal ranges	_____	_____

Check if Completed		Responsible Party	Notes

Instrument Logs for Each Instrument

☐ Purchase date _____ _____

☐ Model and serial numbers _____ _____

☐ Warranties _____ _____

☐ Manufacturer's name and phone number _____ _____

☐ Technical service rep's name/phone number _____ _____

☐ Sales rep's name and phone number _____ _____

☐ Record of each time instrument is serviced _____ _____

Quality Control

☐ Date received and opened on all perishables, reagent log _____ _____

☐ Corrective action log _____ _____

☐ Levy-Jennings graphs with Westgard evaluation each week _____ _____

☐ Mean, CV, SD, evaluated monthly _____ _____

☐ Temperature and humidity logs, if necessary _____ _____

☐ Logs for temps _____ _____

Test Tracking System—Requisitions, Records, Reports: Quality Assurance

☐ QA checklist with monthly evaluation _____ _____

☐ Three levels of QC each day patient tests are run _____ _____

☐ Instrument calibration every 6 months or with each new lot of reagent _____ _____

☐ Routine maintenance performed and documented as needed _____ _____

☐ Consultation/interpretation of results as needed (documented) _____ _____

☐ Generation of test report with tech signature _____ _____

Check if Completed		Responsible Party	Notes

Test Tracking System—Requisitions, Records, Reports: Quality Assurance (continued)

☐ Correction of errors/follow-up of complaints   _____   _____

☐ Maintain QA records for 2 years   _____   _____

☐ Maintain all laboratory records at least 2 years   _____   _____

☐ Keep all instrument set-up records forever   _____   _____

☐ Remedial action policies and procedures   _____   _____

OSHA Standards for Bloodborne Pathogens

☐ Exposure control plan   _____   _____

☐ Universal precautions for all   _____   _____

☐ Offer immunization for hepatitis B   _____   _____

☐ Sharps containers, work practice controls, hand washing   _____   _____

☐ Postexposure evaluation and follow-up— retain records   _____   _____

☐ Appropriate warning labels, training   _____   _____

Miscellaneous

☐ Posted critical values and linearities   _____   _____

☐ Lab director's signature on all manuals   _____   _____

☐ Lab director's specified personnel duties/ responsibilities   _____   _____

☐ Post licenses (personnel and laboratory)   _____   _____

☐ Normal values   _____   _____

☐ Safety manual or section in procedure manual   _____   _____

☐ Protective clothing, gloves, masks, eye protection, face shields   _____   _____

☐ Fire extinguisher charged and inspected on annual basis; employees trained on use of fire blanket   _____   _____

Check if Completed		Responsible Party	Notes

Miscellaneous (continued)

☐ Lids on centrifuges _____ _____

☐ MSDS book _____ _____

☐ Sink _____ _____

☐ Written fire control plan and posted emergency escape route _____ _____

☐ "No smoking" signs posted around flammable liquids _____ _____

☐ Written plan of action for emergencies _____ _____

☐ Exclusive use of refrigerators for chemicals and blood storage _____ _____

Preparation for Recertification CLIA

Please have available the following for review by surveyors at the time of the survey.

Check if Completed		Responsible Party	Notes
☐	Policy and procedure manuals	_____	_____
☐	Specimen collection procedures	_____	_____
☐	Specimen labeling and processing procedures	_____	_____
☐	Step-by-step performance of all testing procedures, including any applicable calculations	_____	_____
☐	Step-by-step performance on instrument calibration and maintenance, including frequency of performance	_____	_____
☐	Equipment range of reportable patient tests	_____	_____
☐	Quality control policies and procedures	_____	_____
☐	Remedial action to be taken when controls are not acceptable	_____	_____
☐	Limitations in testing methodologies, including interfering substances	_____	_____
☐	Normal values	_____	_____
☐	Panic values and established procedures for reporting critical values	_____	_____
☐	Description of course of action to be taken if a test system becomes inoperable	_____	_____
☐	Evidence that the director has reviewed, signed, and dated the manual	_____	_____
☐	Manufacturer's equipment manuals	_____	_____
☐	Personnel records, including education, experience, and copy of applicable licenses	_____	_____

Check if Completed		Responsible Party	Notes
☐	Written description of personnel responsibilities	_____	_____
☐	Safety information	_____	_____
☐	Proficiency testing records and/or proof of enrollment	_____	_____
☐	Examples of test requisitions and accession records, etc	_____	_____
☐	Examples of patient test reports	_____	_____
☐	Written quality assurance (QA) protocol and documentation of OA activities	_____	_____
☐	Procedure for referral of specimens to reference laboratories	_____	_____
☐	Quality control instrument calibration, maintenance records (including temperature records), and manufacturer's insert	_____	_____
☐	Client services manuals, if applicable	_____	_____
☐	Current state laboratory license posted (for recertification survey only)	_____	_____
☐	Current state laboratory personnel licenses posted (as applicable)	_____	_____
☐	Current CLIA certificate available for review	_____	_____

Reporting Laboratory and Test Results to Patients

Patient: _____

Date of test: _____

Routing Slip for Test Results

☐   Normal result: call patient

☐   Normal result: do not call patient

☐   Abnormal result: call, say _____

☐   Abnormal result: Physician will call

☐   Schedule office visit to discuss with patient

☐   Schedule repeat test in _____ (indicate time)

☐   Instructions or comments to patient

_____

_____

_____

☐   Patient called   Date: _____   By: _____

Physician's initials: _____

chapter 7

Health Insurance Portability and Accountability Act

The Health Insurance Portability and Accountability Act (HIPAA) of 1996 is comprehensive legislation that mandated the promulgation of rules for the standardization of health care claims and their submission, as well as privacy, security, unique identifiers, and electronic signature standards. There are three major purposes of HIPAA: (1) to protect and enhance the rights of consumers by providing them access to their health information and controlling the inappropriate use of that information; (2) to improve the quality of health care in the United States by restoring trust in the health care system among consumers, health care professionals, and the multitude of organizations and individuals committed to the provision of care; and (3) to improve the efficiency and effectiveness of health care provision by creating a national framework for health privacy protection that builds on efforts by states, health systems, individual organizations, and individuals.

To comply with the regulations associated with HIPAA, medical practices have adjusted and more tightly controlled their use of patient information. Practices are required to provide patients with notices of privacy and the general ways in which patient data will be used in the practice. Insurance plans have been required by HIPAA to adopt a standardized code set or standardized nomenclature, which currently are the Current Procedural Terminology (CPT) and *International Classification of Diseases, Ninth Revision, Clinical Modification* (ICD-9-CM). In addition, HIPAA provides that if a billing service decides to terminate its services, its data can be transferred to another billing service system without loss of valuable data.

Data communicated by electronic media are standardized. If patient demographic (registration) information, data on the patient encounter form, and data on the billing or claim form were given in the same format as on the Centers for Medicare & Medicaid Services (CMS) 1500 form, substantial money and time could be saved in training. The transfer of data from a billing service that is terminating its service to another billing service also saves time and money and preserves data.

There are training requirements with HIPAA. The employer is responsible within 1 month of a person's employment and annually thereafter to provide education on the rules and guidelines. Certain aspects of employee information are also protected by HIPAA. The forms, checklists, and templates in this chapter are designed to assist medical practices in complying with HIPAA provisions.

Tools for Starting a Practice

Number	Title	Purpose	Notes
07001	Form for Authorized Release of Information From Office or Another Entity	To authorize the release of information for purposes requested by a physician's office from another covered entity	This form gives patients the opportunity to authorize or refuse the disclosure of specific information from one entity to another.
07002	Form for the Authorized Use and Disclosure of Individually Identifiable Information	To authorize the use and disclosure of health care information that can be associated with a specific person or purpose.	To be used in circumstances where normal authorization is insufficient.
07003	Form for the Authorized Use and Disclosure of Information for Physician's Office	To authorize the use and disclosure of information by a practice	This form is used for the same purpose of Tool 07004 but you can be more specific with whom and what is to be disclosed.
07004	Form for Authorization to Release Information to Process Payment	To authorize the practice to release information needed for payment to the insurance company or other payer	This authorization language can be inserted at the bottom of any billing form.
07005	Form for a Budget for HIPAA Compliance Program	To identify the budget needed for HIPAA compliance	This form can be used to help a practice determine the budget for HIPAA compliance.
07006	Form to Obtain Consent to Use and Disclose Health Information	To provide consent for the use and disclosure of health information for treatment, payment, and health care operations	This form is for patients to read and sign, acknowledging understanding of the use of personal data. For the Notice of Information Practices, see Tool 07010.
07007	Template for an Employee Quiz on HIPAA: Privacy Compliance	To assess employee knowledge about HIPAA	Answers. True: questions 1, 2, 4, 6–10, 12, 13, and 15–20. False: questions 3, 5, 11, and 14.
07008	Form for a HIPAA Privacy Regulation Gap Analysis	To list the privacy regulation gap	Use this form to help your practice develop its HIPAA compliance program.
07009	Checklist for the Implementation of HIPAA Privacy and Security Provisions	To assess compliance with the privacy and security provisions of the administrative simplification section of HIPAA	The checklist should be completed to provide identified able steps that have been completed and what still needs to be completed.

Number	Title	Purpose	Notes
07010	Template for a Notice of Information Practices	To notify patients how their protected health information may be used and disclosed and that they can file a complaint if they believe their privacy rights have been violated	This notice describes how information about you may be used and disclosed and how you can gain access to this iinformation.
07011	Template for a Notice of Privacy Practices	To notify patients how medical information may be used and disclosed, how they can gain access to the information, and how they can file complaints if they believe their privacy rights have been violated	Notice must be posted where anyone can see it and a hard copy needs to be made available upon request.
07012	Form for Scheduling Completion of HIPAA Compliance Program	To develop a schedule for compliance with HIPAA	A form to help you set a time schedule for completing you compliance program.
07013	Checklist for Transaction Code Set Rule Compliance	To develop a plan for complying with the transaction code set rule	Use this checklist to assist in implementing your new policies and procedures.
07014	Form for Verification of Information Released	To document the release of medical record information	To be used in the office that released the records to track who released them, to whom, and in which way.

Authorization for Release of Information for Purposes Requested by Physician's Office From Another Covered Entity

I, _____, hereby authorize [Name of Covered Entity disclosing information] to disclose the following protected health information to [Name of Practice]:

[Specifically describe the information to be disclosed, including, but not limited to, meaningful descriptors such as date of service, type of service provided, level of detail to be released, origin of information, etc]

This protected health information is being used or disclosed to carry out treatment, payment, and/or health care operations of [Name of Practice] in the following manner:

[Describe how protected health information will be used to carry out treatment, payment, and/or health care operations purposes.]

This authorization shall be in force and effect until [specify date or event that relates to the patient or the purpose of the use or disclosure], at which time this authorization to use or disclose this protected health information expires.

I understand that I have the right to revoke this authorization, in writing, at any time by sending such written notification to [Name of Privacy Contact] at [office address or e-mail address]. I understand that a revocation is not effective to the extent that [Name of Practice] has relied on the use or disclosure of the protected health information.

I understand that information used or disclosed pursuant to this authorization may be subject to redisclosure by the recipient and may no longer be protected by federal or state law.

[Name of Practice] will not condition my treatment, payment, enrollment (if applicable) in a health plan, or eligibility for benefits on whether I provide authorization for the requested use or disclosure.

I understand that I have the right to refuse to sign this authorization.

_____   _____
Signature of Patient or Personal Representative   Date

_____
Name of Patient or Personal Representative

_____
Description of Personal Representative's Authority

Authorization for the Use and Disclosure
of Individually Identifiable Health Information

I hereby authorize the use or disclosure of my individually identifiable health information as described below. I understand that the information I authorize a person or entity to receive may be redisclosed and no longer protected by federal privacy regulations.

1. Persons/organizations authorized to use or disclose the information: _____

    _____

    _____

2. Persons/organizations authorized to receive the information: _____

    _____

    _____

3. Specific description of information that may be used/disclosed: ___ _____

    _____

    _____

Items 4-6 apply only if the practice is requesting the information for its own uses and disclosures.

4. The information will be used/disclosed for the following purposes: _____

    _____

    _____

5. I understand that this authorization is voluntary and that I may refuse to sign this authorization. My refusal to sign or my revocation of this authorization will not affect my ability to obtain treatment; receive payment; or eligibility for benefits unless allowed by law.

6. The person/organization authorized to use/disclose the information will receive compensation for doing so.
    ☐ Yes   ☐ No

7. I understand that I may inspect or copy the information used or disclosed.

8. I understand that I may revoke this authorization at any time by notifying the person/organization providing the information in writing, except to the extent that:
    a. Action has been taken in reliance on this authorization; or
    b. This authorization is obtained as a condition for obtaining insurance coverage or other law provides the insurer with the right to contest a claim under the policy.

9. This authorization expires on/upon [insert applicable date or event].

_____   _____
Signature of Patient or Patient's Representative   Date

_____   _____
Printed Name of Patient or Patient's Representative   Relationship to Patient or Authority to Act for Patient

Authorization for Use or Disclosure of Information
for Purposes Requested by Physician's Office

I, _____ , hereby authorize [Name of Practice] to (check those that apply):

☐ Use the following protected health information, and/or
☐ Disclose the following protected health information to [Name of entity to receive information]:

[Specifically describe the information to be used or disclosed, including, but not limited to, meaningful descriptors such as date of service, type of service provided, level of detail to be released, origin of information, etc.]

This protected health information is being used or disclosed for the following purposes:

[List specific purposes.]

This authorization shall be in force and effect until [specify date or event that relates to the patient or the purpose of the use or disclosure], at which time this authorization to use or disclose this protected health information expires.

I understand that I have the right to revoke this authorization, in writing, at any time by sending such written notification to [Name of Privacy Contact] at [office address or e-mail address]. I understand that a revocation is not effective to the extent that [Name of Practice] has relied on the use or disclosure of the protected health information.

I understand that information used or disclosed pursuant to this authorization may be subject to redisclosure by the recipient and may no longer be protected by federal or state law.

[Name of Practice] will not condition my treatment, payment, enrollment in a health plan, or eligibility for benefits (if applicable) on whether I provide authorization for the requested use or disclosure.

I understand that I have the right to:
- Inspect or copy the protected health information to be used or disclosed as permitted under federal law (or state law to the extent the state law provides greater access rights)
- Refuse to sign this authorization

[Insert the following sentence if applicable: The use or disclosure requested under this authorization will result in direct or indirect remuneration to the [Name of Practice] from a third party.]

_____   _____
Signature of Patient or Personal Representative   Date

_____
Name of Patient or Personal Representative

_____
Description of Personal Representative's Authority

Authorization to Release Information

I hereby authorize [insert practice name] to release any information required in the course of my examination or treatment as requested by my insurance company (payer of medical benefits) to process payment on my behalf.

_____   _____
Patient's Signature   Date

Budget for HIPAA Compliance Program

Item	Amount
Attend HIPAA Training	$ _____
Consulting Costs	$ _____
Legal Costs	$ _____
Equipment Costs	$ _____
IT/Computer/Software Costs	$ _____
Insurance Costs	$ _____
Miscellaneous/Other Costs	$ _____

Consent to the Use and Disclosure of Health Information for Treatment, Payment, or Health Care Operations

I understand that as part of my health care, [Facility Name] originates and maintains health records describing my health history, symptoms, examination and test results, diagnoses, treatment, and any plans for future care or treatment. I understand that this information serves as:

☐ A basis for planning my care and treatment
☐ A means of communication among the many health professionals who contribute to my care
☐ A source of information for applying my diagnosis and surgical information to my bill
☐ A means by which a third-party payer can verify that services billed were actually provided
☐ A tool for routine health care operations, such as assessing quality and reviewing the competence of health care professionals.

I understand and have been provided with a *Notice of Information Practices* that provides a more complete description of information uses and disclosures. I understand that I have the right to review the notice before signing this consent. I understand that the medical practice reserves the right to change its notice and practices and before implementation will mail a copy of any revised notice to the address I have provided. I understand that I have the right to object to the use of my health information for directory purposes. I understand that I have the right to request restrictions as to how my health information may be used or disclosed to carry out treatment, payment, or health care operations and that the medical practice is not required to agree to the restrictions requested. I understand that I may revoke this consent in writing, except to the extent that the medical practice has already taken action in reliance thereon.

☐ I request the following restrictions to the use or disclosure of my health information.

_____

_____

_____   _____
Signature of Patient or Legal Representative   Date

☐ Accepted   ☐ Denied

_____   _____   _____
              Signature   Title   Date

HIPAA: Privacy Compliance

Employee Name: _____   Date: _____

1.	The HIPAA Privacy Rule ensures that the medical information a patient shares with physicians, hospitals, and others who provide and pay for health care is protected.	☐ True	☐ False
2.	A covered entity includes health care providers, health plans, health care clearinghouses, and business associates with access to patient records.	☐ True	☐ False
3.	Oral information given by a patient to a covered entity is not covered by HIPAA rules.	☐ True	☐ False
4.	HIPAA is about the use and disclosure of protected health information (PHI).	☐ True	☐ False
5.	You are **never** permitted to use or disclose PHI without authorization or agreement from the individual patient.	☐ True	☐ False
6.	PHI is disclosed when it is being shared, examined, applied, or analyzed.	☐ True	☐ False
7.	An authorization form includes the patient signature and should also have an expiration date.	☐ True	☐ False
8.	PHI is generally limited to the minimum amount of information required to get the job done.	☐ True	☐ False
9.	The Patients' Privacy Notice must be available to patients in print and displayed at the site of service.	☐ True	☐ False
10.	A Patients' Privacy Rights must be received at the time of initial service, if patient condition makes that possible.	☐ True	☐ False
11.	The Privacy Rule does not restrict use and disclosure.	☐ True	☐ False
12.	After you receive a signed authorization, the patient can decide to revoke it.	☐ True	☐ False
13.	You can use/disclose PHI without patient agreement to report victims of abuse, neglect, or domestic violence.	☐ True	☐ False
14.	PHI related to minors is controlled solely by the state.	☐ True	☐ False
15.	The Privacy Rule gives patients the right to request a history of nonroutine and routine disclosures.	☐ True	☐ False
16.	The Privacy Rule gives patients the right to take action if their privacy is violated.	☐ True	☐ False
17.	Covered entity administration must ensure that contracts with business associates comply with the Privacy Rule.	☐ True	☐ False
18.	If you violate the Privacy Rule, HIPAA can levy civil and criminal penalties.	☐ True	☐ False
19.	The responsibility to ensure that HIPAA regulations are followed lies only with the HIPAA compliance officer.	☐ True	☐ False
20.	The Department of Health and Human Services is required to give you assistance if there is a rule you do not understand.	☐ True	☐ False

ACKNOWLEDGMENT OF TRAINING

I have attended the training session and/or read the training information about HIPAA. I have completed and passed the comprehensive quiz at the conclusion of my training.

_____   _____
Signature of Employee   Date

_____   _____
Signature of Trainer   Date

HIPAA Privacy Regulation Gap Analysis

1. Has your practice designated a privacy officer to carry out the requirements of the HIPAA privacy standards?

    ☐ Yes   ☐ No

    A.   If yes, specify who: _____

    B.   If no, your practice needs to designate a privacy officer as soon as possible, and the privacy officer must be responsible for the development and implementation of your practice's HIPAA compliance program and its policies and procedures.

    C.   Name of privacy officer: _____

    D.   Date completed: _____

2. Does your practice need to designate other staff members or employees as part of its HIPAA compliance committee or team?

    ☐ Yes   ☐ No

    A.   Depending on the size of your practice, your practice may need to designate additional individuals and participants to assist the privacy officer with the development and implementation of the practice's HIPAA compliance program. Examples of staff members and employees who may need to be on your practice's HIPAA compliance committee or team include your practice's office manager, MIS director, billing department director or representative, medical records department chairperson or representative, possibly one of your practice's physicians, your director of or representative from your quality assurance department, and your practice's risk manager, as applicable.

    B.   List the names of your practice's compliance committee: _____

    _____

    _____

    _____

    C.   Date completed: _____

3. Is there an employee or staff member in your practice designated as the contact person to receive and handle complaints or grievances from patients concerning your practice's privacy practices and handling of patients' medical records and protected health information?

    ☐ Yes   ☐ No

    A.   HIPAA requires that your practice designate an individual who will handle complaints and grievances from patients concerning privacy issues and matters. **Recommendation:** Your practice should select an employee or staff member who not only has good working knowledge of the HIPAA privacy regulations and applicable state law, but also has strong interpersonal and "people" skills and who is skilled in handling questions and complaints from patients.

    B.   Name of grievance/complaint contact person: _____

    C.   Date completed: _____

4. Has your practice developed a policy and procedure for the handling of patient grievances and complaints concerning your practice's privacy practices and its handling of patient medical records and protected health information?

    ☐ Yes   ☐ No

    A. HIPAA requires your practice to develop a written policy and procedure for the handling of grievances and complaints.

    B. Date completed: _____

5. Has your practice developed a Notice of Privacy Practices?

    ☐ Yes   ☐ No

    A. HIPAA requires your practice to provide patients with a Notice of Privacy Practices. **Recommendation:** Refer to the template Notice of Privacy Practices (Tool 07011).

    B. Date completed: _____

6. Is your practice familiar with HIPAA's prerequisites for its Notice of Privacy Practices and the documentation required for such Notices? Additionally, has your practice developed written policies and procedures concerning the use of its Notice of Privacy Practices?

    ☐ Yes   ☐ No

    A. **Recommendation:** Your practice will need to implement policies and procedures concerning Notices of Privacy Practices and ensure that your practice's staff and employees are trained in the use of the Notice.

    B. Date completed: _____

7. Has your practice identified all of the ways it receives patient medical records and protected health information into the practice?

    ☐ Yes   ☐ No

    A. As part of your practice's gap analysis, one of the first tasks your practice should complete is to identify all of the ways in which it receives patient medical records and protected health information from other parties, as well as what parties the practice receives patient medical records and protected health information from.

    Recommendation: Identify who your practice receives such information from.

    (1) Other physicians: _____
    (2) Hospitals: _____
    (3) Nursing homes/long-term care facilities: _____
    (4) Health insurers/managed care companies: _____
    (5) Patients: _____
    (6) Patients' family members or legal representatives: _____
    (7) Pharmacies: _____
    (8) Durable medical equipment companies: _____
    (9) Medical device manufacturers: _____
    (10) Other: _____

    B. Your practice should also identify the ways in which it receives such information

    (1) Telephone: _____
    (2) Facsimile: _____
    (3) Verbally: _____
    (4) E-mail: _____
    (5) Other electronic format: _____
    (6) Paper: _____
    (7) CD-ROM: _____

(8)   Other: _____

C.   Date completed: _____

8.   Has your practice identified all of the ways in which it uses and stores patient medical records and protected health information?

☐ Yes   ☐ No

A.   As part of your practice's gap analysis, your practice should identify all the ways in which it uses patient medical records and protected health information, as well as the methods and ways in which it stores such information. **Recommendation:** Your practice should identify all of the ways in which it uses and stores the information, including:

B.   Uses

(1)   Treatment: _____

(2)   Payment: _____

(3)   Health care operations: _____

(4)   Employment determinations: _____

(5)   Clinical research trials: _____

(6)   Marketing: _____

(7)   Coordination of benefits: _____

(8)   Claims inquiries: _____

(9)   Quality assurance: _____

(10) Other: _____

C.   Storage methods

(1)   Electronic medical records/computer: _____

(2)   On-site storage: _____

(3)   Off-site storage: _____

(4)   Filing cabinets/shelves: _____

(5)   Third-party storage company: _____

(6)   Other: _____

D.   Date completed: _____

9.   Has your practice identified all of the ways, and to whom, it discloses patient medical records and protected health information?

☐ Yes   ☐ No

A.   Your practice needs to identify all of the individuals and entities to which it discloses patient medical records and protected health information. **Recommendation:** Use the following checklist to identify the individuals and entities:

(1)   Other treating physicians and health care practitioners: _____

(2)   Hospitals: _____

(3)   Nursing homes/long-term care facilities: _____

(4)   Pharmacies: _____

(5)   Clinical laboratories: _____

(6)   Diagnostic imaging centers: _____

(7)   Patients: _____

(8)   Patients' family members or legal representatives: _____

(9)   Health insurers/managed care companies: _____

(10) Quality assurance organizations: _____

(11) Attorneys: _____

(12) Accountants: _____

(13) Transcriptionists: _____

(14) Courier services: _____

(15) Patients' employers: _____

(16) Document storage companies: _____

(17) Document destruction companies: _____

(18) Practice management consultants: _____

(19) Assisted living facilities: _____

(20) Adult daycare centers: _____

(21) Ambulatory surgery centers: _____

(22) Case managers: _____

(23) Medical device manufacturers: _____

(24) Durable medical equipment companies: _____

(25) Hospices: _____

(26) Home health agencies: _____

(27) Computer hardware or software vendors: _____

(28) Pharmaceutical companies: _____

(29) Medical researchers: _____

(30) Other (Recommendation): _____

B. Your practice should identify all of the ways in which it releases patient medical records and protected health information to other individuals and entities. **Recommendation:** Use the following checklist to identify the ways in which your practice releases such information:

(1) Verbally: _____

(2) Facsimile: _____

(3) E-mail: _____

(4) Telephone: _____

(5) Paper/hand deliver: _____

(6) Other: _____

C. Date completed: _____

10. Has your practice conducted initial, basic training on the HIPAA privacy requirements for your staff and employees?

☐ Yes ☐ No

A. **Recommendation:** As your practice is developing and implementing its compliance program, it should familiarize its employees with the basic concepts established by the HIPAA privacy regulations. For example, your employees should have some basic training as to what constitutes protected health information; how they should handle it; what they can do to help your practice identify how it receives, uses, stores, and discloses patient medical records and protected health information; and how your practice will use its Notice of Privacy Practices, Consents, and Authorizations. A brief initial training session with designated employees and staff members of approximately 1 hour would probably be sufficient.

B. Date completed: _____

11. Has your practice made a distinction between consents and authorizations and how they are going to be developed, implemented, and used by your practice?

☐ Yes ☐ No

Date completed: _____

12. Does your practice fully understand the patient rights developed by HIPAA?

    ☐ Yes   ☐ No

    Date completed: _____

13. Are your staff and employees familiar with the circumstances in which your practice may disclose a patient's protected health information without a consent or authorization?

    ☐ Yes   ☐ No

    A. **Recommendation:** You should provide training to your staff and employees on the circumstances in which your practice may release a patient's protected health information without a consent or authorization.

    B. Date completed: _____

14. Does your Notice of Privacy Practices notify patients as to how uses and disclosures will be made of their protected health information without their consent or authorization?

    ☐ Yes   ☐ No

    A. Date completed: _____

15. Is your practice currently documenting medical record disclosures for its patients?

    ☐ Yes   ☐ No

16. Does your practice have a written policy and procedure concerning responding to criminal, civil, and administrative subpoenas?

    ☐ Yes   ☐ No

    A. **Recommendation:** Your practice should develop and implement a written policy and procedure on how to handle and respond to subpoenas.

    B. Date completed: _____

17. Does your practice have a written policy and procedure concerning the release of patient medical record information or protected health information by telephone?

    ☐ Yes   ☐ No

    A. **Recommendation:** Your practice should implement a written policy and procedure concerning the release of patient medical record information and protected health information via telephone.

    B. Date completed: _____

18. Does your practice have a written policy and procedure concerning the use of faxes to receive or send patient medical record information or protected health information?

    ☐ Yes   ☐ No

    A. **Recommendation:** Your practice should develop a written policy and procedure concerning the receipt or disclosure of patient medical record information and protected health information via faxes.

    B. Date completed: _____

19. Does your practice have a written policy and procedure concerning the release of patient medical record information or protected health information by e-mail?

    ☐ Yes   ☐ No

    A. **Recommendation:** Your practice should develop a written policy and procedure concerning the release of patient medical record information and protected health information via e-mail.

    B. Date completed: _____

20. Do your physicians, staff and employees recognize and understand the various areas of superconfidential information under state law?

☐ Yes ☐ No

A. **Recommendation:** As part of your practice's training program, your physicians, employees and staff should be made aware of the superconfidential information under state law.

B. Date completed: _____

21. Is your practice able to identify all the situations in which a business associate contract must be in place?

☐ Yes ☐ No

A. **Recommendation:** Your practice should **immediately** identify all potential Business Associates with which it must have a business associate contract.

B. Date completed: _____

22. Does your practice maintain its medical records and patient files for at least 6 years?

☐ Yes ☐ No

For 7 years?

☐ Yes ☐ No

23. Does your practice manage its medical records and patient files in a way that allows for patients to inspect and/or have access to or release of their medical record information and files?

☐ Yes ☐ No

A. **Recommendation:** Your practice should develop policies and procedures for these subject areas.

B. Date completed: _____

24. Are your physicians, staff, and employees aware of your practice's obligations and rights if patients request amendments to their medical records or protected health information?

☐ Yes ☐ No

25. If you answered "yes" to the previous question, does your practice have a policy and procedure in place for handling amendments to patient medical records?

☐ Yes ☐ No

A. **Recommendation:** Your practice should develop written policies and procedures concerning amendments to patient medical records and protected health information.

B. Date completed: _____

26. Do your physicians, employees, and staff have a complete understanding of the concept of minimum necessary disclosure for various disclosures of protected health information?

☐ Yes ☐ No

A. **Recommendation:** Your practice should develop a written policy and procedure for minimum necessary disclosures.

B. Date completed: _____

27. Are your physicians, staff, and employees aware of the 18 identifiers set forth by HIPAA that can be used to deidentify protected health information?

☐ Yes ☐ No

A. **Recommendation:** Your practice should not only develop a written policy and procedure concerning these areas, but also ensure that its physicians, employees, and staff are familiar with and understand the 18 identifiers.

B. Date completed: _____

28. Does your practice currently hold or conduct any training sessions for its physicians, employees, and staff concerning HIPAA, patient medical record confidentiality, and protected health information?

☐ Yes ☐ No

29. Does your practice maintain records of the individuals who attend training sessions on HIPAA, patient medical record confidentiality, and protected health information?

☐ Yes ☐ No

30. Does your practice have a policy and procedure designed to handle breaches of patient confidentiality?

☐ Yes ☐ No

A. **Recommendation:** Your practice should develop and implement a policy and procedure concerning how to handle a breach in patient confidentiality.

B. Date completed: _____

31. Does your practice have a policy and procedure for handling grievances and patient complaints?

☐ Yes ☐ No

A. **Recommendation:** Your practice should develop a written policy and procedure for handling patient grievances and complaints concerning their protected health information.

B. Date completed: _____

32. Does your Notice of Privacy Practices include notice to patients that they have the right to file a complaint with the Secretary of the US Department of Health and Human Services (HHS)?

☐ Yes ☐ No

33. Does your practice's Notice of Privacy Practices enumerate the process by which patients may file a complaint with the Secretary of HHS?

☐ Yes ☐ No

34. Are your practice's physicians, employees, and staff encouraged to identify areas of potential noncompliance with HIPAA?

☐ Yes ☐ No

35. Does your practice have a policy and procedure in place concerning restriction of access to protected health information?

☐ Yes ☐ No

A. **Recommendation:** Your practice needs to develop written policies and procedures that clearly delineate when physicians, employees, and staff may have access to patients' medical records and protected health information.

B. Date completed: _____

36. Does your practice's physical security protection include:

A. Equipment being raised off the floor if there is a danger of flooding:

☐ Yes ☐ No

B. Alarm systems in place and operational to alert for possible water damage:

☐ Yes   ☐ No

C. All critical equipment protected by surge protectors or voltage regulators:

☐ Yes   ☐ No

D. Smoke-, heat-, or flame-activated detectors installed and tested:

☐ Yes   ☐ No

E. Sufficient fire extinguishers available:

☐ Yes   ☐ No

F. Storage of paper and electronic medical records and protected health information in fireproof containers:

☐ Yes   ☐ No

G. Automatically activated sprinkler system:

☐ Yes   ☐ No

H. A sprinkler system that automatically turns off electricity before the sprinklers are activated:

☐ Yes   ☐ No

I. If possible, water pipes routed away from computer equipment:

☐ Yes   ☐ No

J. Emergency shut offs that are easily accessed:

☐ Yes   ☐ No

K. Only one door that accesses each secure area where patient medical records and protected health information are stored:

☐ Yes   ☐ No

L. A layout that ensures that all persons entering secure areas must pass by a receptionist or staff member:

☐ Yes   ☐ No

M. Key locks to secure areas replaced by programmed locks:

☐ Yes   ☐ No

N. Visitors signed in and out of secure areas and provided with badges:

☐ Yes   ☐ No

O. Visitors to secure areas accompanied by staff members:

☐ Yes   ☐ No

P. A security alarm:

☐ Yes   ☐ No

Q. Electrical wiring closets that are not shared with other functions and that are secured by heavy doors with programmed locks:

☐ Yes   ☐ No

37. Has your practice designated an employee or staff member to maintain and update its written policies and procedures?

☐ Yes   ☐ No

38. Are your practice's written policies and procedures managed in a way that would allow employees and staff members access to them for at least 6 years?

☐ Yes   ☐ No

39. Has your practice developed date-sensitive standards for all documentation in written or electronic format?

☐ Yes   ☐ No

40. Has your practice educated its employees and staff on its HIPAA implementation timeline?

   ☐ Yes   ☐ No

   Date completed: _____

41. Is your practice familiar with the applicable state law concerning confidentiality of medical records?

   ☐ Yes   ☐ No

   A. **Recommendation:** Your practice should conduct training for its physicians, employees and staff concerning applicable state laws regarding confidentiality of medical records.

   B. Date completed: _____

42. Has your practice trained its physicians, staff, and employees on their responsibility and duties to cooperate with and respond to investigations by HHS and other government agencies concerning patient medical records and protected health information?

   ☐ Yes   ☐ No

   Date completed: _____

43. Have each of your practice's physicians, staff, and employees signed a confidentiality agreement?

   ☐ Yes   ☐ No

   Date completed: _____

44. Does your practice have a written contract with each business associate with which it does business?

   ☐ Yes   ☐ No

   Date completed: _____

45. Does your practice have a policy and procedure for responding to patients who request an accounting of your practice's disclosures of the patients' protected health information?

   ☐ Yes   ☐ No

   A. **Recommendation:** Your practice needs to develop a written policy and procedure for tracking such disclosures and providing an accounting to patients of such disclosures.

   B. Date completed: _____

46. Has your practice filed an extension request or its compliance report for HIPAA's Standard Transaction and Code Set Requirements?

   ☐ Yes   ☐ No

   Date completed: _____

47. Has your practice reviewed its medical malpractice/professional negligence, general comprehensive liability and other insurance policies to determine if they provide coverage and defense for HIPAA violations, state or federal agency investigations concerning patient medical record confidentiality issues, and/or private or civil lawsuits alleging breach of privacy claims?

   ☐ Yes   ☐ No

   A. **Recommendation:** Contact your practice's insurance broker or agent and ask whether your practice's insurance policies cover such violations, investigations, and/or lawsuits.

   B. Date completed: _____

Implementation of the Privacy and Security Provisions
of the Administrative Simplification Section of HIPAA

Check if Completed		Responsible Party	Notes

☐   Designate the person or persons responsible for the development and implementation of the practice's privacy and security policies.

☐   Convene a staff meeting to inform everyone of the importance of these federal standards and that this is an opportunity for them to provide input into changes or modifications made to the processes currently in effect in the office(s).

☐   Begin the assessment of the practice, including the applicable areas listed in this checklist. Remember to document all of your efforts.

Assess the audit trail process currently available in your current computer system.

☐   Is there a strict system in place for log-on identification?

☐   Does the system log out after a short time and require password entry again?

☐   Is this password unique?

☐   Does this password allow the user to access only a predetermined set of information and services? (Remember to provide very limited access to the records of employees who are also patients of the practice.)

☐   Is the list of passwords maintained by one person (system administrator)?

☐   Is there a system in place for immediate termination of an individual's password and access rights?

☐   Does your system identify and restrict access to an individual who does not have authorized access?

Check if Completed		Responsible Party	Notes
☐	Is there a discipline policy to address sharing of passwords and other breeches in the log-in system?	_____	_____
	☐ Is this policy strictly enforced?	_____	_____
	☐ Is it enforced consistently for all members of the organization, regardless of their position, including physicians, owners, etc?	_____	_____
☐	Is there a means to create emergency log-on identification?	_____	_____
☐	Is there a system/policy to create onetime access for such users as temporary employees or auditors?	_____	_____
☐	Is there a system in place that allows for monitoring the procedures to ensure and document compliance?	_____	_____
☐	Does your system have the capability to generate reports that will document the practice's compliance, such as exception reports?	_____	_____
☐	Do you have a policy in place to generate reports of compliance of the computer system, including random sampling and exception reports?	_____	_____
	☐ Do you track a variety of data elements, such as time/date access, system entry of persons without appropriate access, geographic location (different offices), diagnosis code indicators highlighting access into patient chart/information with specific "sensitive" diseases, and access into the records of employees who are patients of the practice records?	_____	_____
☐	If there is a suspected breach in the security or privacy elements of your computer system, can your computer system perform a search function to access an individual's activity or individual patient record access?	_____	_____
☐	Is there a backup system in place for your entire computer system?	_____	_____
☐	Is the backup system schedule followed and documented?	_____	_____

Check if Completed		Responsible Party	Notes
☐	Are the backup files kept off-site in a secure place?	_____	_____
	☐ Is this location secure? Who has access to this location?	_____	_____
☐	Does the practice/organization use personal digital assistants (PDAs) for recording data?	_____	_____
☐	Do these PDAs have password protection?	_____	_____
☐	Do these PDAs have a backup and purging schedule?	_____	_____
☐	Is this schedule maintained and documented?	_____	_____
☐	Are you using the Internet to transmit data?	_____	_____
☐	Although there is no such thing as absolute security, do you document the efforts you have made to maintain the integrity and privacy of your transmitted data?	_____	_____
☐	Have you developed a written disaster recovery plan for all emergencies and/or system failures?	_____	_____

Perform a walk-through of your entire office area and look for items such as:

☐	Is there a patient sign-in sheet that is left on a counter or that is easily seen by other patients who enter the office?	_____	_____
☐	Can any computer screens be seen by anyone approaching the reception desk or checkout area?	_____	_____
☐	Can any computer screens be seen by unauthorized persons anywhere else in the office?	_____	_____
☐	Do patients have to check out in an area that others can easily overhear protected health information, such as diagnosis, ordered tests, etc?	_____	_____
☐	Is the fax machine accessible to unauthorized persons walking by, and do they have the ability to pick up or read an incoming or outgoing fax message?	_____	_____

Check if Completed		Responsible Party	Notes

Perform a walk-through of your entire office area and look for items such as: (continued)

☐ Is the copy machine accessible to an unauthorized person walking by who may pick up or read information being copied?

☐ Are there files accessible that an unauthorized person could either read or remove from the office?

☐ Are there locks on doors for the filing area, or are the file cabinets locked?

☐ Are patient records/files lying on counters or desks that can be seen by patients or other unauthorized persons?

☐ Does your fax machine use film that could be read if not destroyed?

☐ Are patient records removed from the office?

☐ Are patient records transported in a locked container?

☐ Is there a HIPAA-compliant process in place to transfer patient records and/or information to requesting entities such as other health care providers, insurance companies, attorneys?

☐ Does this policy/process address the minimum necessary requirements under HIPAA?

Have you identified the persons and entities considered business associates?

☐ Transcription vendors

☐ Billing companies

☐ Collection agencies

☐ Webmaster/Web site administrator

☐ Document management

☐ Coding vendors

☐ Computer hardware and software vendors

Check if Completed		Responsible Party	Notes

Have you identified the persons and entities considered business associates? (continued)

☐ Computer repair vendors _____ _____

☐ Clearinghouse vendor _____ _____

☐ Maintenance personnel _____ _____

☐ Landlord _____ _____

☐ Legal counsel _____ _____

☐ Third-party payers _____ _____

☐ Locum tenens workers _____ _____

☐ Temporary staffing agencies _____ _____

☐ Risk-management consultants _____ _____

☐ Compliance and audit vendors _____ _____

☐ Joint venture partners _____ _____

☐ Waste management vendors _____ _____

☐ Any other entity who has potential access to protected health information _____ _____

☐ Have you reviewed your present contracts/agreements for HIPAA compliance? _____ _____

☐ After performing the assessment, have you developed an action plan to comply with the HIPAA rules? _____ _____

☐ Have you developed a HIPAA-compliant authorization form for all patients to read and sign? _____ _____

☐ Have you developed a HIPAA-compliant Notice of Information Practices? _____ _____

☐ Is this displayed in an area for all patients to read? _____ _____

☐ Is the Notice of Information Practices given to any new and existing patients who request it? _____ _____

Check if Completed		Responsible Party	Notes
☐	Have you developed a business associate agreement or amendment to your current contracts?	_____	_____
☐	Have you developed a written policy and procedure manual (or incorporated them into your corporate compliance program) regarding the elements of the HIPAA compliance program?	_____	_____
☐	Have you established a training schedule?	_____	_____
☐	Have you established a HIPAA compliance record-keeping system?	_____	_____
☐	Have you established a set of policies and procedures to maintain up-to-date information regarding existing and future HIPAA standards?	_____	_____

Another assessment tool that may be helpful to your practice or organization is to have someone unknown to the staff make an appointment and become a new patient of the practice. Have this person perform an assessment of the features you have implemented and record any failures in the system. This person should have enough knowledge to attempt to breach the security and privacy functions of the organization, but should also have signed a confidentiality statement before being permitted to perform this assessment. If staff members are informed that this assessment method is being used, they will be aware that security procedures are being monitored.

Another way to gather information about the security of the practice or organization is to have a meeting with staff members and brainstorm about areas they believe are vulnerable. Areas or types of threats to address are areas found in the assessment checklist and also the following areas.

Check if Completed		Responsible Party	Notes
☐	Human error (erasures, accidental damage, deliberate acts, improper disposal of paper and disks, etc)	_____	_____
☐	Nature (fire, water, lightning, earthquake, etc)	_____	_____
☐	Technical (lack of backup, system failure, virus, loss of power, etc)	_____	_____
☐	Deliberate (unauthorized disclosure, modification)	_____	_____

Once you have performed your assessment, the next step is to address the vulnerabilities of your organization. These include any areas found in your assessment and the following areas.

Check if Completed		Responsible Party	Notes

Physical security (environmental, installation)

☐   Area access controls   _____   _____

☐   Accountability controls   _____   _____

☐   Equipment enclosures, lockdown, locks   _____   _____

☐   Fire protection systems   _____   _____

☐   Encryption   _____   _____

☐   System security software, mainframes, networks, etc.   _____   _____

Technical controls (ie, what data may be accessed or removed from original location to remote areas via file transfer, uploads to the Internet, jump drives, etc.)

☐   Disaster recovery   _____   _____

Operational security (the who, what, where, when, why, and how often actions)

☐   Standard operational policies and procedures   _____   _____

☐   Accountability controls   _____   _____

☐   Nondisclosure contracts and confidentiality statements   _____   _____

☐   Regularly scheduled training   _____   _____

☐   Definitions of levels of information security   _____   _____

☐   Need-to-know basis   _____   _____

☐   Backing up data   _____   _____

☐   Audit trails   _____   _____

Notice of Information Practices

*This notice describes how information about you may be used and disclosed and
how you can gain access to this information. Please review it carefully.*

1. [Facility Name] may use and disclose protected health information for treatment, payment, and health care operations. Examples of these include, but are not limited to, requested preschool, life insurance, or sports physicals, and referral to nursing homes, foster care homes, home health agencies, and/or referral to other providers for treatment. Payment examples include, but are not limited to, insurance companies for claims including coordination of benefits with other insurers and collection agencies. Health care operations include, but are not limited to, internal quality control and assurance including auditing of records.

2. [Facility Name] is permitted or required to use or disclose protected health information without the individuals' written consent or authorization in certain circumstances, such as for public health requirements and court orders.

3. [Facility Name] will not make any other use or disclosure of a patient's protected health information without the individual's written authorization. Such authorization may be revoked at any time. Revocation must be written.

4. [Facility Name] may at times contact the patient to provide appointment reminders or information regarding treatment alternatives or other health-related benefits and services that may be of interest to the individual patient.

5. [Facility Name] will abide by the terms of this notice or the notice currently in effect at the time of the disclosure.

6. [Facility Name] reserves the right to change the terms of its notice and to make new notice provisions effective for all protected health information that it maintains.

7. [Facility Name] will provide each patient with a copy of any revisions of its Notice of Information Practices at the time of the next visit or at the last known address if there is a need to use or disclose any protected health information of the patient. Copies may also be obtained at any time at our offices.

8. Any person/patient may file a complaint to the medical practice and to the Secretary of Health and Human Services if they believe their privacy rights have been violated. To file a complaint with the practice, please contact the privacy officer at the following address and/or telephone number [insert area code and telephone number]. All complaints will be addressed, and the results will be reported to the corporate compliance officer.

9. It is [Facility Name]'s policy that no retaliatory action will be made against any individual who submits or conveys a complaint of suspected or actual noncompliance of the privacy standards.

10. The name, title, and telephone number of a person in the office to contact for further information are [Name and Title] at [insert area code and telephone number].

The Effective Date: [insert date, which cannot be earlier than the date on which the notice is printed or otherwise published]

Notice of Privacy Practices

Effective Date: [insert date]

THIS NOTICE DESCRIBES HOW MEDICAL INFORMATION ABOUT YOU MAY BE USED AND DISCLOSED AND HOW YOU CAN GET ACCESS TO THIS INFORMATION. PLEASE REVIEW IT CAREFULLY.

If you have any questions about this notice, please contact [insert contact information].

WHO WILL FOLLOW THIS NOTICE

This notice describes our practice's privacy practices and that of:

- Any physician or health care professional authorized to enter information into your medical chart.
- All departments and units of the practice.
- All employees, staff, and other office personnel.
- All these individuals, sites, and locations follow the terms of this notice. In addition, these individuals, sites, and locations may share medical information with each other or with third-party specialists for treatment, payment, or office operations purposes described in this notice.

OUR PLEDGE REGARDING MEDICAL INFORMATION

We understand that medical information about you and your health is personal. We are committed to protecting medical information about you. We create a record of the care and services you receive at our office. We need this record to provide you with quality care and to comply with certain legal requirements. This notice applies to all of the records of your care generated by our office.

This notice will tell you about the ways in which we may use and disclose medical information about you. We also describe your rights and certain obligations we have regarding the use and disclosure of medical information.

We are required by law to:

- Ensure that medical information that identifies you is kept private;
- Give you this notice of our legal duties and privacy practices with respect to medical information about you; and
- Follow the terms of the notice that is currently in effect.

HOW WE MAY USE AND DISCLOSE MEDICAL INFORMATION ABOUT YOU.

The following categories describe different ways that we use and disclose medical information. Not every use or disclosure in a category will be listed. However, all of the ways we are permitted to use and disclose information will fall within one of the categories.

- **For Treatment.** We may use medical information about you to provide you with medical treatment or services. We may disclose medical information about you to the practice's office personnel who are involved in taking care of you at the office or elsewhere. We also may disclose medical information about you to people outside our office who may be involved in your care after you leave the office, such as family members or others we use to provide services that are part of your care, provided you have consented to such disclosure. These entities include third-party physicians, hospitals, nursing homes, pharmacies, and clinical laboratories with whom the office consults or makes referrals.
- **For Payment.** We may use and disclose medical information about you so that the treatment and services you receive at our office may be billed to and payment may be collected from you, an insurance company, or a third party. For example, we may need to give your health plan information about procedures you received at the office so your health plan will pay us or reimburse you for the services. We may also tell your health plan about a treatment you are going to receive to obtain prior approval or to determine whether your plan will cover the treatment.
- **For Health Care Operations.** We may use and disclose medical information about you for medical office operations. These uses and disclosures are necessary to run our office and make sure that all of our patients receive quality care. For example, we may use medical information to review our treatment and services and to evaluate the performance of our staff in caring for you. We may also combine medical information about many patients to decide what additional services the office should offer, what services are not needed, and whether certain new treatments are effective. We may also disclose information to our physicians, staff, and other office personnel for review and learning purposes.
- **Appointment Reminders.** We may use and disclose medical information to contact you as a reminder that you have an appointment for treatment or medical care at the office.

- **Treatment Alternatives.** We may use and disclose medical information to tell you about or recommend possible treatment options or alternatives that may be of interest to you.
- **Health-Related Benefits and Services.** We may use and disclose medical information to tell you about health-related benefits or services that may be of interest to you.
- **Individuals Involved in Your Care or Payment for Your Care.** We may release medical information about you to a friend or family member who is involved in your medical care, provided you have consented to such disclosure. We may also give information to someone who helps pay for your care. In addition, we may disclose medical information about you to an entity assisting in a disaster relief effort so that your family can be notified about your condition, status, and location.
- **As Required By Law.** We will disclose medical information about you when required to do so by federal, state, or local law.
- **To Avert a Serious Threat to Health or Safety.** We may use and disclose medical information about you when necessary to prevent a serious threat to your health and safety or the health and safety of the public or another person. Any disclosure, however, would only be to someone able to help prevent the threat.

SPECIAL SITUATIONS

- **Health Oversight Activities.** We may disclose medical information to a health oversight agency for activities authorized by law. These oversight activities include, for example, audits, investigations, inspections, and licensure. These activities are necessary for the government to monitor the health care system, government programs, and compliance with civil rights laws.
- **Lawsuits and Disputes.** If you are involved in a lawsuit or a dispute, we may disclose medical information about you in response to a court or administrative order. We may also disclose medical information about you in response to a subpoena, discovery request, or other lawful process by someone else involved in the dispute, but only if efforts have been made to tell you about the request or to obtain an order protecting the information requested.
- **Law Enforcement.** We may release medical information if asked to do so by a law enforcement official:
  - In response to a court order, subpoena, warrant, summons, or similar process;
  - To identify or locate a suspect, fugitive, material witness, or missing person;
  - About the victim of a crime if, under certain limited circumstances, we are unable to obtain the person's agreement;
  - About a death we believe may be the result of criminal conduct;
  - About criminal conduct at the office; and
  - In emergency circumstances to report a crime; the location of the crime or victims; or the identity, description, or location of the person who committed the crime.
- **Coroners, Medical Examiners, and Funeral Directors.** We may release medical information to a coroner or medical examiner. This may be necessary, for example, to identify a deceased person or determine the cause of death. We may also release medical information about patients of the office to funeral directors as necessary to perform their duties.

YOUR RIGHTS REGARDING MEDICAL INFORMATION ABOUT YOU

You have the following rights regarding medical information we maintain about you:

- **Right to Inspect and Copy.** You have the right to inspect and copy medical information that may be used to make decisions about your care. To inspect and copy medical information that may be used to make decisions about you, you must submit your request in writing to [insert information]. If you request a copy of the information, we may charge a fee for the costs of copying, mailing, or other supplies associated with your request. We may deny your request to inspect and copy in certain very limited circumstances.
- **Right to Amend.** If you feel that medical information we have about you is incorrect or incomplete, you may ask us to amend the information. You have the right to request an amendment for as long as the information is kept by or for our office.

  To request an amendment, your request must be made in writing and submitted to [insert information]. In addition, you must provide a reason that supports your request.

  We may deny your request for an amendment if it is not in writing or does not include a reason to support the request. In addition, we may deny your request if you ask us to amend information that:

  - Was not created by us, unless the person or entity that created the information is no longer available to make the amendment;
  - Is not part of the medical information kept by or for our office;
  - Is not part of the information that you would be permitted to inspect and copy; or
  - Is accurate and complete.

- **Right to an Accounting of Disclosures.** You have the right to request an "accounting of disclosures." This is a list of the disclosures we made of medical information about you.

  To request this list or accounting of disclosures, you must submit your request in writing to [insert information]. Your request must state a time period, which may not be longer than 6 years and may not include dates before [insert dates]. Your request should indicate in what form you want the list (for example, on paper, electronically). The first list you request within a 12-month period will be free. For additional lists, we may charge you for the costs of providing the list. We will notify you of the cost involved, and you may choose to withdraw or modify your request at that time before any costs are incurred.

- **Right to Request Restrictions.** You have the right to request a restriction or limitation on the medical information we use or disclose about you for treatment, payment, or health care operations. You also have the right to request a limit on the medical information we disclose about you to someone who is involved in your care or the payment for your care, like a family member or friend. For example, you could ask that we not use or disclose information about a surgery you had. ***We are not required to agree to your request.*** If we do agree, we will comply with your request unless the information is needed to provide you emergency treatment.

  To request restrictions, you must make your request in writing to [insert information]. In your request, you must tell us (1) what information you want to limit; (2) whether you want to limit our use, disclosure, or both; and (3) to whom you want the limits to apply, for example, disclosures to your spouse.

- **Right to Request Confidential Communications.** You have the right to request that we communicate with you about medical matters in a certain way or at a certain location. For example, you can ask that we only contact you at work or by mail.

  To request confidential communications, you must make your request in writing to [insert information]. We will not ask you the reason for your request. We will accommodate all reasonable requests. Your request must specify how or where you wish to be contacted.

- **Right to a Paper Copy of This Notice.** You have the right to a paper copy of this notice. You may ask us to give you a copy of this notice at any time. Even if you have agreed to receive this notice electronically, you are still entitled to a paper copy of this notice.

  You may obtain a copy of this notice at our Web site, [insert site address].

  To obtain a paper copy of this notice, [insert information].

CHANGES TO THIS NOTICE

We reserve the right to change this notice. We reserve the right to make the revised or changed notice effective for medical information we already have about you as well as any information we receive in the future. We will post a copy of the current notice in the office. The notice will contain on the first page, in the top right-hand corner, the effective date. In addition, each time you register, we will offer you a copy of the current notice in effect.

COMPLAINTS

If you believe your privacy rights have been violated, you may file a complaint with the office or with the Secretary of the Department of Health and Human Services. To file a complaint with our practice, contact **[insert the name, title, and phone number of the contact person or office responsible for handling complaints. This should be the same person or department listed on the first page as the contact for more information about this notice.]** All complaints must be submitted in writing.

You will not be penalized or retaliated against for filing a complaint.

OTHER USES OF MEDICAL INFORMATION

Other uses and disclosures of medical information not covered by this notice or the laws that apply to us will be made only with your written permission. If you provide us permission to use or disclose medical information about you, you may revoke that permission, in writing, at any time. If you revoke your permission, we will no longer use or disclose medical information about you for the reasons covered by your written authorization. You understand that we are unable to take back any disclosures we have already made with your permission and that we are required to retain our records of the care that we provided to you.

[Insert Name of Practice]

Acknowledgment of Notice of Privacy Practices

Our Notice of Privacy Practices provides information about how we may use and disclose protected health information about you. You have the right to review our Notice before signing this form. As provided in our Notice, the terms of our Notice may change. If we change our Notice, you may obtain a revised copy by [insert information].

You have the right to request that we restrict how protected health information about you is used or disclosed for treatment, payment, or health care operations. We are not required to agree to this restriction, but if we do, we are bound by our agreement.

By signing this form, you consent to our use and disclosure of protected health information about you for treatment, payment, and health care operations as described in our Notice. You have the right to revoke this consent, in writing, except where we have already made disclosures in reliance on your prior consent.

Patient: _____
                                         (Print)

               _____
                                      (Signature)

Date: _____

Witness: _____

Schedule for Completion of HIPAA Compliance Program

Task	Date
Attend HIPAA Workshop	
Establish Budget	
Complete Gap Analysis	
Develop and Implement Policies and Procedures	
Conduct Employee Training	
File Standard Transactions and Code Sets Extension	
Complete Business Associate Contracts	
Complete Implementation of HIPAA Compliance Program	
Compliance Deadline	

Transaction Code Set Rule Compliance

Check if Completed		Responsible Party	Notes
☐	Designate one person to be responsible for this set of HIPAA rules.	_____	_____
☐	Download and review the implementation guidelines from http://aspe.hhs.gov/ or http://www.wpc-edi.com/hipaa. You may have up to a 50% increase in information that must be transmitted that you are currently not transmitting.	_____	_____
☐	Contact your practice management/billing software vendor to review the necessary changes to comply with these rules. Remember, the provider, not the software vendor, is responsible for transmitting the necessary information.	_____	_____
☐	Create a timeline for implementation of new data entry information. Remember that you will have to coordinate your conversion with any trading partners, such as clearinghouses, Medicare, Medicaid, etc.	_____	_____
☐	Perform testing with each of the entities with which you transmit information.	_____	_____
☐	Develop a set of policies and procedures necessary to ensure compliance with this rule.	_____	_____
☐	Develop a training schedule for all staff involved in the implementation of the Transaction Code Set Rules	_____	_____

Verification of Information Released

Name and Title of Person Who Released Records: _____

Please describe which records were released: _____

How was the information transferred?

☐ **By US Mail**

_____   _____
Date Sent   Certification No., if Certified

☐ **By Fax**

_____   _____
Date Faxed   Fax Number

☐ **By Courier**

_____   _____
Date of Pick Up   Courier Name

☐ **In Person**

_____   _____
Date of Pick Up   Name

Verification of identification performed?   ☐ Yes   ☐ No

chapter 8

Quality Improvement and Risk Management

Although quality care has always been a goal of medical practices, attention was dramatically focused on quality when the Institute of Medicine released its various reports on the state of health care in the United States. Providers, payers, regulators, and patients are more aware of quality issues.

Ensuring quality care involves many activities, and terms used include quality improvement (QI), quality assurance (QA), and quality control (QC). Although the definitions of the terms vary somewhat, the goal of QI, QA, and QC is common: to effectively provide the care needed by patients, when they need it. The steps in ensuring quality care include identifying the care that is needed (on the basis of accurate diagnostic data and diagnoses), determining how to provide the care most effectively (on the basis of, for example, patient and community needs, services available, and outcome data), and determining whether the care was effective.

Physicians and staff can identify areas of the practice that are effective and real and potential problems. For example, if outcome data show that a previously effective drug no longer works for a number of patients, additional data are needed to identify the real problem (eg, the type of medication, the reason for use, prescribing patterns of individual physicians, instructions given to patients, adherence of patients to instructions, and pharmacies used by the patients). Simply changing prescriptions might solve individual patient problems but could overlook a deeper issue, such as a mislabeled drug in a pharmacy used by several affected patients.

Despite measures to ensure quality care, mistakes can still happen, and patients can still have unexpected or unique reactions. Therefore, ensuring quality care means also having a nonpunitive means to identify and correct errors and of communicating with patients openly and honestly about errors. The risk management literature and literature on error reduction include a multitude of articles and tools that would be helpful to medical practices.

Patients, physicians, and all office staff need to be involved in efforts to ensure quality care. The forms in this chapter are designed to help obtain the data needed.

Tools for Quality Improvement and Risk Management

Number	Title	Purpose	Notes
08001	Form for a Patient Complaint	To provide patients with an means to describe a complaint and suggest resolution	Aggregate data about patient complaints can be used to identify the need for changes in the practice, such as revising scheduling procedures to reduce wait times or including information on billing forms to help patients understand the bill.
08002	Form for a Patient Satisfaction Survey	To monitor patient satisfaction with a practice	The aggregate data from the surveys can be used for an overall evaluation of the practice, and individual comments might provide helpful suggestions for improvement in problem areas.
08003	Form for a Patient Satisfaction Survey: In-Office Surgeries and Procedures	To monitor patient satisfaction in a surgical center	The data obtained from this form assist in the ongoing data collection for the office's quality improvement process.
08004	Form for QI Physician Peer Review	To identify required areas in medical records and determine the appropriateness of diagnoses and treatments	An ongoing quality improvement program includes a method for physician peer review. A reviewing physician may be another physician in the group or if a solo practice an arrangement can be made with a physician's colleague.
08005	Form for QI Laboratory Training Documentation	To document laboratory training	The documentation of training can serve as one basis for differentiating whether a problem is lack of knowledge or skill or related to systems and processes.
08006	Form for a Quality Assurance Problem Identification Report	To document a problem and the action taken	When these reports are collected over time, the data can be used to identify trends and consistent problems and to evaluate the effectiveness of the resolution and actions taken. The form can be completed by any member of the QI team or can be used to summarize the findings of any of the other QI monitoring reports.
08007	Form for a Patient Satisfaction Survey	To determine patient satisfaction with services	

Patient Complaint

Date: _____

Please describe any problem you experienced.

_____

_____

_____

_____

_____

_____

_____

How can we help resolve it?

_____

_____

_____

_____

_____

_____

_____

Name of Patient:_____

Information Provided/Taken by: _____

Referred to:_____

Resolved by:_____

Patient Notified of Action: _____

Date: _____

Patient Satisfaction Survey

How would you rate the following on a scale from 1 to 10 (1 being *poor* and 10 being *excellent*)?

Physician care	1	2	3	4	5	6	7	8	9	10
Nursing care	1	2	3	4	5	6	7	8	9	10
Front office personnel	1	2	3	4	5	6	7	8	9	10
Office environment: waiting rooms, treatment areas, etc	1	2	3	4	5	6	7	8	9	10
Billing/collection procedures	1	2	3	4	5	6	7	8	9	10
Length of time the physician spends with you	1	2	3	4	5	6	7	8	9	10
Physician's handling of your telephone calls	1	2	3	4	5	6	7	8	9	10
Physician's patience and interest in your problem	1	2	3	4	5	6	7	8	9	10

Additional Suggestions:

_____

When you last called our office, did you find our staff to be helpful and thorough?

☐ Yes, very much   ☐ Somewhat   ☐ No, not at all

Comment:

_____

How long did you wait in the waiting room?

☐ Fewer than 15 minutes   ☐ 15 to 30 minutes   ☐ More than 30 minutes

Comment:

_____

How long did you wait in the treatment room before the physician entered?

☐ Fewer than 15 minutes   ☐ 15 to 30 minutes   ☐ More than 30 minutes

Comment:

_____

What do you consider to be the strengths of this office?

_____

How could this office improve its services to you? Are there additional programs and services *not* currently available that we should add? Please specify.

_____

Please feel free to give any further comments.

_____

Name, address, and phone number are optional. We welcome signed and unsigned forms.

_____

[Client Name]
Patient Satisfaction Survey

The care of our patients is our chief concern, and we are continually striving to improve the service. You can help us by answering the following confidential questionnaire. Thank you for your help in assuring high quality of care for our future patients. Please rate your satisfaction below:

5 = Excellent   4 = Very good   3 = Good   2 = Fair   1 = Poor   NA = Not applicable

Overall Impressions

Ease of being admitted	5	4	3	2	1	NA
Waiting time in the reception area	5	4	3	2	1	NA
Privacy needs were met	5	4	3	2	1	NA
Staff treated you with courtesy and respect	5	4	3	2	1	NA

Care by Your Physician

Available to talk with you as needed	5	4	3	2	1	NA
Clearly answered all your questions	5	4	3	2	1	NA

Care by the Staff

Sensitive to your needs	5	4	3	2	1	NA
Answered your questions satisfactorily	5	4	3	2	1	NA
Competent	5	4	3	2	1	NA

Preparation for Discharge

Received clear and detailed discharge instructions	5	4	3	2	1	NA
All questions answered before discharge	5	4	3	2	1	NA
Understood how to contact physician, if needed	5	4	3	2	1	NA

Overall

Quality of care and services received:	5	4	3	2	1	NA

I would recommend this facility to family and friends: ☐ Yes   ☐ No

In what ways could we improve the care and services at the surgery center?

_____

_____

Patient Name (OPTIONAL): _____   Date: _____

Thank you for giving us your opinions. We will use this information in summarizing
*overall patient satisfaction and for quality improvement purposes **only**.*

QUALITY IMPROVEMENT PHYSICIAN PEER REVIEW

[insert Client Name]

Month: _____   Year: _____

Total procedures done in: _____   Month: _____

Physician: _____

Answer each question for each medical record number with yes (Y), no (N), or not applicable (N/A).	Medical Record Number											
History and physical are adequate on the basis of the chief complaint?												
Diagnoses are appropriate for the findings in the H&P?												
Diagnostic procedures are appropriate on the basis of the diagnosis?												
Treatment is consistent with the working diagnosis?												
Patient outcome is recorded?												
Complications are identified and documented?												
Procedure is one that is included in the physician's scope of practice as identified by his/her privileges?												
Refer to physician of record for comment?												
Requires action by medical director?												

Signature of Physician Reviewer: _____   Date: _____

Comments: _____

Created: [Date]

[electronic file name and path]

Laboratory Training Documentation

Employee Name: _____

Note: Date each item as it is completed.

	Begin	6 Months	1 Year	Comments
GENERAL				
Calibration Protocols and Procedures				
Critical Values				
Equipment Maintenance				
Normal Ranges				
Quality Control				
Read and Sign Test Procedure				
Read Procedure Manual				
Read Product Insert				
Reagent Stability/Storage				
DIRECT OBSERVATION				
Function Checks				
Instrument Maintenance				
Patient Preparation				
Specimen Rejection				
Specimen Collection				
Specimen Handling/Labeling				
Specimen Preservation/Storage				
Specimen Processing				
Specimen Testing				
MONITORING				
Recording/Reporting				
REVIEW				
Maintenance Records				
Quality Control Records				
Test Results/Worksheet				
ASSESSMENT OF TEST PERFORMANCE				
Assessment of Problem Solving Skills				
External Proficiency Testing				
Internal Blind Testing				
Previously Analyzed Specimen				
Troubleshooting				
OTHER TECHNICAL TRAINING				
Hazardous Waste Disposal				
MSDS Workbook				

Trainer: _____ **Begin** Date: _____

Trainer: _____ **6 Months** Date: _____

Trainer: _____ **1 Year** Date: _____

Quality Assurance Problem Identification Report

Investigation

Physician _____   Initials: _____

Chart No.: _____

Patient: _____

Identification: _____

Problem

_____

_____

_____

_____

_____

Resolution/Action Taken

_____

_____

_____

_____

_____

[insert Practice Name]
Patient Satisfaction Survey

The care of our patients is our chief concern, and we are continually striving to improve the service. You can help us by answering the following confidential questionnaire. Thank you for your help in ensuring high quality of care for our future patients. Please rate your satisfaction.

	Poor	Fair	Good	Very Good	Excellent	Unknown or Not Applicable
Overall Impressions	☐	☐	☐	☐	☐	☐
Office environment cheerful	☐	☐	☐	☐	☐	☐
Waiting time in the reception area	☐	☐	☐	☐	☐	☐
Privacy needs were met	☐	☐	☐	☐	☐	☐
Staff treated you with courtesy and respect	☐	☐	☐	☐	☐	☐
Care by Your Physician	☐	☐	☐	☐	☐	☐
Available to talk with you as needed	☐	☐	☐	☐	☐	☐
Clearly answered all your questions	☐	☐	☐	☐	☐	☐
Care by the Nurse and Staff	☐	☐	☐	☐	☐	☐
Sensitive to your needs	☐	☐	☐	☐	☐	☐
Answered your questions satisfactorily	☐	☐	☐	☐	☐	☐
Competent	☐	☐	☐	☐	☐	☐
Overall Quality of Care and Services Received	☐	☐	☐	☐	☐	☐

When you last called our office, did you find our staff to be helpful and thorough?   ☐ YES   ☐ NO

How long did you wait in the waiting room?   _____

How long did you wait in the treatment room before the physician entered? _____

What do you consider to be the strengths of this office? _____

_____

In what ways could we improve the care and services in this practice? _____

_____

I would recommend this facility to family and friends.   ☐ YES   ☐ NO

Your Name (optional): _____   Date: _____

Thank you very much for giving us your opinions. We will use this information in summarizing overall patient satisfaction and for quality improvement purposes only.

chapter 9

Clinical Processes and Forms

Documentation of care provided is essential to an effective medical practice. Documentation indicates the quality and findings of assessment, including laboratory and radiologic test results; the diagnoses considered and selected; the plan for treatment and the actual treatment performed; medications prescribed; and follow-up, including an assessment of the outcomes of therapeutic measures. It also indicates special needs of patients and unique characteristics. It provides information for tracking a patient's progress over time and provides information to be used by other providers, should the need arise. Patients and family members might seek documentation if a hereditary disease is found.

In addition to the benefits to quality care provided by quality documentation, the documentation also is used by regulatory agencies for various functions, by courts, and by third-party payers.

Physicians who practice with high populations of nursing home, care facilities, or workers' compensation injuries require to provide more multidiscipline oversight of those patients.

The forms, template, and checklist in this chapter are designed to aid in documentation related to clinical care in both the hospital nursing facilities and home care.

Tools for Clinical Processes

Number	Title	Purpose	Notes
09001	Form for DRG Documentation Guidelines	To illustrate a form for review of a record for DRG 239 for pathological fractures and musculoskeletal and connective tissue malignancy	Sections I and II are completed concurrently.
09002	Form for an Interdisciplinary Case Management Communication Tool: Nursing Home Patients Care	To record interdisciplinary communication about one or more issues	When your practices have patients who receiving care in an extended care facility, skilled nursing facility, or convalescent home. This form can be used to track that process of your patient population.
09003	Template for a Medical Procedure Consent	To document consent for a medical procedure	

Number	Title	Purpose	Notes
09004	Form for a Patient Discharge: Choice of Continuing Care	To inform patients or responsible parties of the physician's orders for continuing care after discharge from the hospital, identify patient choices of service providers, and obtain consent to contact the service providers	
09005	Form for Patient Medication Education	To inform patients about how and when to take medications	In addition to this information, patients also should know what to expect from the medication (eg, side effects, adverse effects, when to call about effects, how long before therapeutic effects are usually noticed, what to do if a dose is missed, whether it is okay to abruptly discontinue taking the medication, the need to take all antibiotics even if feeling well). Patients' understanding of this information and anticipated or possible barriers to adherence to the regimen should be assessed. For example, if a patient cannot take a medication every 6 hours as prescribed, a plan should be developed with the patient for a workable schedule that still permits effectiveness.
09006	Form for Patient Rehabilitation Progress	To monitor the progress of a patient's rehabilitation	
09007	Form for Photographic Wound Documentation	To document patient wounds photographically and descriptively	
09008	Checklist for Preoperative Procedures	To provide a checklist of items required before an operative procedure can begin in the physicians office.	This form is applicable to practices in which surgical procedures are routinely performed, such as plastic surgery practices, and outpatient surgical centers; however, it can be adapted to the needs of any practice.
09009	Forms for Special Orthotic/Prosthetic Certification	To certify that a patient needs these devices	This tool includes two forms, one for patients with conditions that require, diabetic shoes, orthotics, or other prosthetic devices, to request certification of need and one for the physician treating the patient.
09010	Form for a Family Conference Report	To document a conference with family	The physician should use this form to have record of a meeting with the patient's family regarding care and follow-up.

DRG Documentation Guidelines

Readmission Rate:	Patient Name:
Denial for DRG:	MR No.:

DRG No.: 239
Pathological Fractures and Musculoskeletal and Connective Tissue Malignancy

	Done	Date of Activity		Notes
		Discussed With Physician	Discussed With Nursing	

Section I: Admission—Hospital Course (Documentation Requested by Physician)

	Done	Discussed With Physician	Discussed With Nursing	Notes
Document clinical indications for admission; examples: ■ Evidence of injury on X ray ■ Presence of deformity, local swelling and discoloration, and soft tissue damage ■ Pain ■ Loss of function ■ Restriction of posture and movement				
Document the plan for admission.				
Document *all* comorbid conditions. Be specific. Examples: ■ Diabetes: document type and if controlled or uncontrolled ■ Cancer: document origin of malignancy ■ Anemia: document reason for (due to blood loss) and whether acute or chronic				
Relate symptoms to diagnoses; examples: ■ Anemia related to renal failure ■ CHF secondary to valve replacement				
Review and document results of laboratory and diagnostic tests; appropriate orders to correct abnormal findings.				
Document daily progress notes to address response to therapy. Document the etiology/cause of the fracture. Document site of the fracture, and note whether pathological or traumatic.				
Write discharge order when there is clinical and hemodynamic stability of systems.				
Discharge summary to include discharge diagnosis, disposition of patient, and follow-up visit plan.				
Document medical necessity of drug therapies.				

Created: [Date]

[electronic file name anc path]

Patient Name:				
Readmission Rate:				
Denial for DRG:	MR No.:			

DRG Documentation Guidelines

DRG No.: 239
Pathological Fractures and Musculoskeletal and Connective Tissue Malignancy

	Done	Date of Activity		Notes
		Discussed With Physician	Discussed With Nursing	
Section II: Case Management				
Document diagnoses in order of importance. Discharge summary should include all findings, all diagnoses, and pertinent laboratory findings with a detailed discussion of the hospital course.				
Note that consultant reports are reviewed, opinion is considered and is part of treatment plan per physician orders.				
Ensure admission to appropriate level of care.				
Initiate discharge planning: ▪ Assess need for rehab facility or home care options ▪ Assess psychosocial needs; initiate appropriate referrals ▪ Evaluate need for durable medical equipment				
Review laboratory and diagnostic test results.				
Discuss expected goals/outcomes with the physician, patient/family, and other ancillary department caregivers.				
Observe daily progress and patient response to treatment, including: ▪ Skin and wound management ▪ Pain management ▪ Neurovascular status ▪ Nutritional status: intake and output ▪ Activity and exercise enhancement ▪ Readiness for patient/family education assessed and initiated by nursing staff				
Facilitate transition to next level of care.				

Date:	
Current Census in Nursing Home:	
Expected Discharges:	
Expected Admissions:	

Staffing

7 am – 7 pm	RN	CNA	UC
7 pm – 7 am	RN	CNA	UC

Issues	Follow up
Patient Care	
Case Management	
Risk Management	
Social Services	
Quality	
Administration	

Confidential report for improvement of nursing facility and patient care. Not part of medical record and not to be used in litigation.

Medical Consent

I, _____, have agreed to the following procedure to be done in the office by [insert physician name], on the day of _____ _____, 20____. The procedure has been fully explained to me, including any benefits and risks.

Name of the procedure: _____

Risks discussed: _____

_____

_____

Person providing information to the patient: _____

_____   _____
Patient Signature   Date

_____   _____
Witness Signature   Date
(cannot be the provider of the surgery)

Choice of Continuing Care

1. You are being discharged from [insert practice name]. Your physician has ordered:

   ☐ Home Health Services   ☐ Nursing Home Services

   ☐ Skilled Nursing/Swing Bed Services   ☐ Assisted Living Center Services

   ☐ Outpatient Therapy Services   ☐ Acute Rehabilitation Services

   ☐ Durable Medical Equipment (DME)   ☐ Other: _____

2. Prior to hospitalization, were you using any of these services?
   ☐ Yes   ☐ No

3. If so, what services were you utilizing before hospitalization, and which ones do you want us to contact with your hospital discharge orders?

	Services Prior to Hospitalization	**Services Chosen to Be Contacted**
☐ Home Health Service	_____	_____
☐ Nursing Home Service	_____	_____
☐ Skilled Nursing/Swing Bed Services	_____	_____
☐ Assisted Living Center Services	_____	_____
☐ Outpatient Therapy Service	_____	_____
☐ Acute Rehabilitation Services	_____	_____
☐ Durable Medical Equipment (DME)	_____	_____
☐ Other	_____	_____

_____

_____

4. Do you feel that you were provided with enough information about available services to make a decision in which you feel comfortable?
   ☐ Yes   ☐ No   ☐ NA (not applicable)

_____   _____
Signature of Patient or Responsible Party   Social Services Representative

_____   _____
Relationship (if Responsible Party)   Date

COMMENTS: _____

_____

_____

5. Discharge information (date, care services, etc.) provided to:

   ☐ Patient: _____

   _____

   ☐ Family/Support Person(s): _____

   _____

   ☐ Physician: _____

   _____

6. Name of continuing care agency: _____

   Information provided to the continuing care agency via:

   ☐ Fax (fax notice to be part of medical record): _____

   ☐ Telephone: _____

   ☐ Packet: _____

   _____

[insert practice name]
Patient Medication Education Sheet

Patient: _____   **Allergies:** _____

Drug	Amount/Frequency	Times							Taken For

Created: [Date]

[electronic file name and path]

ROOM # : _____   ADMIT DATE: _____

Type of Assistance	Dependent	Maximum	Moderate	Minimal	Contact Guard	Standby	Independent
Supine ⬍ Sit							
Sit ⬍ Stand							
Stand pivot transfers							
Wheelchair							
Walking							
Bathing upper body							
Bathing lower body							
Dressing upper body							
Dressing lower body							
Toileting							
Feeding							
Swallowing							

Physical Therapy Devices

Continuous Passive Motion Unit:

Walker: ☐ Standard ☐ Front wheel ☐ Four wheel ☐ Brake extensions ☐ Other: _____

Occupational Therapy Devices

Long-Handled: ☐ Sponge ☐ Shoehorn ☐ Reacher ☐ Sling ☐ Other: _____

Feeding: _____

Swallowing: _____

☐ Room privileges up ad lib   ☐ Floor privileges up ad lib   # of person assist: _____

Created: [Date]

Photographic Wound Documentation

Circle the wound location.

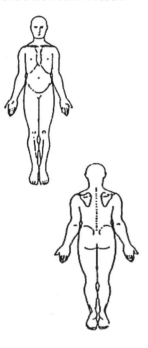

PHOTO	Date	Stage
	Depth	Odor
	Size in centimeters (width × length)	
	Presence or absence of drainage/type	
	Color/Description	
	Signature	
	Photographer	

Circle the wound location.

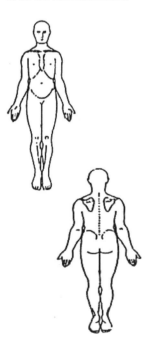

PHOTO	Date	Stage
	Depth	Odor
	Size in centimeters (width × length)	
	Presence or absence of drainage/type	
	Color/Description	
	Signature	
	Photographer	

Preparation for Preoperative Procedures

In preparing procedure records for the next procedural day, the following checklist will be utilized and included within the record for review by the preoperative nurse prior to the procedure. Any items that have been requested but not received should be identified as such.

Check if Completed		Responsible Party	Notes
☐	Summary of Procedures	_____	_____
☐	Pre/Post-Proc Phone Call to Patient or Designee	_____	_____
☐	Preprocedural Instructions	_____	_____
☐	Patient Demographic Sheet	_____	_____
☐	Physician Order Sheet	_____	_____
☐	HIPAA Privacy Notice	_____	_____
☐	History and Physical	_____	_____
☐	Insurance Card Copies	_____	_____
☐	Informed Consent	_____	_____
☐	Adv. Directives Notification	_____	_____
☐	Pre/Post/Intra-Proc Record	_____	_____
☐	Advance Directives Document	_____	_____
☐	Discharge Instructions	_____	_____
☐	Operative Report	_____	_____
☐	Progress Notes	_____	_____
☐	Anesthesia Record	_____	_____
☐	Testing, if ordered; Results Noted	_____	_____
☐	Anesthesia History/Evaluation	_____	_____

All forms required to be present on chart for designated procedure are present as indicated.

_____   _____

Signature   Date

Day of Procedure

_____   ☐ N/A (local anesthesia)

The responsible person listed above will remain in the center during
the procedure and will drive the patient home from the facility.

Patient: _____

Physician: _____

I certify that all of the following statements are true:

- This patient has diabetes mellitus
- This patient has one or more of the following conditions (it is not necessary to specify which apply):
  - History of partial or complete amputation of the foot
  - History of previous foot ulceration
  - History of preulcerative callus formation
  - Peripheral neuropathy with evidence of callus formation
  - Foot deformity
  - Poor circulation
- I am treating this patient under a comprehensive plan of care for his/her diabetes.
- This patient needs special shoes and/or inserts because of his/her diabetes.

This statement care be prepared by the prescriber or supplier but must be reviewed and signed by the certifying physician. The certifying physician must be an MD or DO and not a podiatrist.

Signed: _____

Date: _____

Date: _____

_____
Physician's Name

_____
Address

_____
City   State   Zip Code

Dear Dr. _____:

Your patient, _____, has been seen and treated in our office for diabetic foot problems (ie, vascular, neuropathic, or ulcerative).

I believe that your patient would benefit from special orthotics/prosthetics in order to prevent a worsening of his/her condition.

I would appreciate your signing the attached certification letter so that I may dispense special orthotics/prosthetics. A stamped, return envelope is enclosed for your convenience. Should you have any questions, please do not hesitate to contact my office.

Thank you,

_____
Physician's signature

Enclosures

Family Conference Date: _____   **Time:** _____

Patient Present

☐ Yes   ☐ No   If no, why not? _____

Family Present (list name and relationship)

_____   _____

_____   _____

_____   _____

_____   _____

Summary

Provided/Discussed: ☐ Clinical Update   ☐ Prognosis   ☐ Disposition

_____

_____

_____

_____

_____

_____

Follow-up/Recommendations

_____

_____

_____

_____

_____

Estimated Length of Stay: _____   **Discharge Date:** _____

Signature and Title of Persons Attending

_____   _____

_____   _____

_____   _____

_____   _____

chapter 10

Human Resources and Staff Development

To run a successful practice, staff matched to needs of the practice are essential. Physicians must determine the types of positions needed; how many people are required for each type of position; how employees will be recruited, employed, trained, supervised, compensated, evaluated, and retained; and what the practice can afford in personnel costs.

Matching individual employees to the practice is important. Employees need to be compatible with physicians' styles of interactions. Employees' skills should be complementary. For example, a practice that treats children and adults should seek staff to meet the needs of both groups rather than hiring nurses with only pediatric or adult intensive care experience. To the extent possible, employees who interact frequently should be compatible, and any employees who have contact with patients need effective communication skills.

The tools in this chapter focus primarily on basic employment and orientation and training issues and the proper forms to use for basic employment practices. Chapter 11 provides information more specific to evaluation and compensation, staff development, work relationships, and various forms related to employment.

Tools for Human Resources and Staff Development

Number	Title	Purpose	Notes
10001	Form for an Attendance Record	To record and employee's use of sick leave and vacation time	
10002	Checklist for Manager Training on Gender Bias	To list ways to avoid gender bias in the office	
10003	Form for Mandatory Annual Training Control Log	To document CPR, OSHA, CLIA, domestic violence, and HIPAA training for employees	
10004	Form for a Confidential Employee History	To document personal employee information related to licensure, taxes, and a contact person	

Number	Title	Purpose	Notes
10005	Form for Employee Confidentiality and Security Agreement	To comply with proper employee use of computers	
10006	Template for an Employee Orientation Program	To list the topics and contents of an employee orientation program	
10007	Form for Employment Application	To provide a form for employment application	
10008	Form for an Individual Employee Education Record	To document employee education and meeting attendance	This form also identifies educational requirements, such as safety training.
10009	Form for Sample Interview Questions	To identify potential questions for interviewing job applicants	
10010	Checklist for Information and Forms for New Employees	To provide a checklist for information and forms needed by new employees	This information and forms in this checklist are needed so new employees can be identified and paid and learn about policies and procedures.
10011	Checklist for Payroll Service Outsourcing	To list considerations for outsourcing payroll services	
10012	Checklist for Personnel File	To document employment, health-related, and work-related educational, certification, licensure, and training information for personnel	This form can be used to track various requirements for all employees on monthly and annual bases. May be used to audit contents of personnel files.
10013	Checklist for Personnel Records	To indicate the information that must be retained in personnel records	These records need to be maintained for as long as your state records laws dictate. Consult your individual state record retention rules to determine how long personnel records are to be kept.
10014	Checklist for Recruitment: Converting Applicants to Patients	To list ways to use employee recruitment, interviewing, and hiring practices to recruit patients	
10015	Form for a Time Sheet	To provide a sample time sheet	
10016	Checklist for Employee Confidentiality	To ensure privacy of confidential information of staff members	

Number	Title	Purpose	Notes
10017	Checklist for New Employee Personnel Training	To provide a list of topics and items for consideration when starting a new practice	Also see Tool 10005 for a detailed list of orientation topics.
10018	Checklist for Successful Interviews and Recruitment	To provide suggestions for a successful interview	
10019	Form for Employment Drug Screen Consent	To obtain consent for preemployment drug screening by urine testing	
10020	Form for Leave Request	To provide uniform information when leave is requested by employees	
10021	Form for a Keys Issued Record	To provide record of keys issued	
10022	Form for a Request for Expense Reimbursement	To provide for requests for reimbursement of work-related expenses	
10023	Form for Tuition Assistance	To request tuition assistance	
10024	Form for Workers' Compensation: Notice of Injury	To report a work-related injury	
10025	Forms for Workers' Compensation: Treatment	To document approval of treatment and billing information in a workers' compensation case	For the occupational health information card, use a 5 x 8 index card and file alphabetically by employer (company).

Attendance Record

Employee Name: _____   Employee Number: _____

Pay Period	Sick Leave			Vacation		
	Accrued	Used	Available	Accrued	Used	Available

Gender Bias Training

Check if Completed		Responsible Party	Notes
☐	Avoid stereotyping men and women. Not all men are aggressive or masculine, and not all women are sensitive and sweet.	_____	_____
☐	Sexual harassment can go both ways. Always take it seriously no matter who it is.	_____	_____
☐	Dress codes should be the same for men and women in comparable positions.	_____	_____
☐	Do not assume that men and women have different career goals. All employees should get regular reviews and pay increases.	_____	_____
☐	Do not assign tasks on the basis of gender. Ask yourself whether you would ask a person of the opposite gender to do the same thing.	_____	_____
☐	Do not label or refer to women as "girls" or men as "boys."	_____	_____

Mandatory Annual Training Control Log

Name	Position	Type of Training Control (CPR, OSHA, CLIA, Domestic Violence, or HIPAA)	Certification No. (if required)	Training Date

Employee History
CONFIDENTIAL

_____ _____ _____
Employee Name   Birth Date   Social Security Number

	Date	Exemption
Federal Withholding		
State Withholding		
Other		

_____ _____
Address   Apt #

_____ _____ _____
City   State   ZIP Code

Professional Licenses/Certification	Date Granted	Renewal Date

Training Received	Date

Emergency Contact's Name: _____

Relation to Employee: _____

Telephone: (Day)_____ (Night) _____

_____ _____
Employment Date   Anniversary Date

_____ _____
Termination Date   Reason for Termination

Employee Confidentiality and Security Agreement

I understand that [insert name of practice], for whom I work, has a legal and ethical responsibility to safeguard the privacy of all patients and to protect the confidentiality of patients' health information. In addition, the practice must ensure the confidentiality of its human resources, payroll, fiscal, research, internal reporting, strategic planning, communications, computer systems, and management information (referred to hereafter, along with patient-identifiable health information, as "confidential information").

During the course of my employment at the practice, I understand that I may come into the possession of confidential information. I will access and use this information only when it is necessary to perform my job-related duties in accordance with the practice's privacy and security policies. I further understand that I must sign and comply with this agreement in order to obtain authorization for access to confidential information.

1. I will not disclose or discuss confidential information with others, including family or friends, who do not need to know it.

2. I will not divulge, copy, release, sell, loan, alter, or destroy confidential information except as properly authorized.

3. I will not discuss confidential information where others can overhear the conversation. It is not acceptable to discuss confidential information, even if the patient's name is not used.

4. I will not make unauthorized transmissions, inquiries, modifications, or purging of confidential information.

5. I agree that my obligations under this agreement will continue after termination of my employment, expiration of my contract, or cessation of my relationship with the practice.

6. Upon termination, I will immediately return documents or media containing confidential information to the practice.

7. I understand that I have no right to ownership interest in any information accessed or created by me during my relationship with the practice.

8. I will act in the best interests of the practice and in accordance with its HIPAA compliance program at all times during my relationship with the practice.

9. I understand that violation of this agreement may result in disciplinary action, up to and including termination of employment, suspension and loss of privileges, or termination of authorization to work within the practice, in accordance with the practice's policies.

10. I will only access or use systems or devices I am officially authorized to access and will not demonstrate the operation or function of systems or devices to unauthorized individuals.

11. I understand that I should have no expectation of privacy when using the practice's information systems. The practice may log, access, review, and otherwise use information stored on or passing through its systems, including e-mail, in order to manage systems and enforce security.

12. I will practice good workstation security measures, such as locking up disks when not in use, using screensavers with activated passwords appropriately, and positioning screens away from public view.

13. I will practice secure electronic communications by transmitting confidential information only to authorized entities, in accordance with approved security standards.

14. I will:
    a. Use only my officially assigned user ID and password;
    b. Use only approved licensed software; and
    c. Use a device with virus protection software.

15. I will never:
    a. Share or disclose user IDs or passwords;
    b. Use tools or techniques to break or exploit security measures; or
    c. Connect to unauthorized networks through the systems or devices.

16. I will notify the practice's privacy officer or security officer if my password has been seen, disclosed, or otherwise compromised, and I will report activity that violates this agreement or privacy and security policies and any other incident that could have an adverse effect on confidential information.

By signing this document, I acknowledge that I have read this agreement and agree to comply with all the terms and conditions stated above.

Employee/Physician Signature _____

Employee/Physician Printed Name _____

Date _____

Physical Plant Tour

Physical location of:

- Reception area
- Pre- and postprocedure areas
- Procedural suites
- Locker rooms
- Cleanup and sterilizing areas
- Waiting area
- Examination rooms
- Medication refrigerator
- Break area
- Food refrigerator
- Restrooms

- Hazards substances
- Secured areas for communications
- Computer
- Personnel introductions
- Confidentiality
- Patient relations and handle calls and inquiries
- Dirty utility rooms
- Supply areas
- Tank room
- Traffic flow
- Exits

Manuals

Review of the following manuals, program, and plans:

- Policies and procedures manuals—both administrative and clinical
- Bloodborne pathogen and hazard communication
- TB exposure control
- Quality improvement program
- HR manual

- MSDS manual
- Forms manual
- Equipment instruction manual
- Agreements/contracts manual
- Certifications/licensure manual
- Job descriptions manual

Communications

- Line of authority—review of organizational chart
- Telephone and intercom system

Equipment

- In-service education on all equipment located in the office
- Competency requirements for using equipment
- Documentation and troubleshooting of problems with equipment
- Equipment availability

Function of the Procedural Team (if Applicable)

- Physician
- Anesthesia personnel
- Circulator

- Medical assistant
- Pre- and postprocedure nurses
- Receptionist

Principles of Aseptic Technique

- Procedural gowning and gloving (self-closed method)
- Procedural gowning and gloving of others
- Procedural draping
- Infection control

- Preparation and maintenance of procedural area
- Procedural scrubbing routine
- Medical asepsis

Sterilization: Types and Principles

- Autoclave utilization and maintenance
- Sterilization principles

Procedural Case

- Organization of room
- Handling of sterile articles—as circulator
- Procedural fields—nonsterile and sterile areas
- Supplies and instruments

- Physician preference cards and maintenance, if applicable
- Location of clean and sterile items

Patient Medical Record

- Contents of medical record
- Policies and procedures outlining the organization of the medical record
- Required tests, history, and physical, etc
- Informed consent

- Forms specific to the practice
- Guidelines for completion
- Authentication policy for identifying patients
- Confidentiality

Preprocedure Routine

- Preparation of patient
- Medications to be administered
- Initiation of IV access

- Preprocedure identification
- Medical record checked for appropriate contents and verified

Procedural Suite Routine

- Obtaining of appropriate items necessary for specific procedure
- Opening of sterile supplies and instruments
- Patient arrival in suite
- Patient and procedural site identification by physician, anesthesia, and circulator
- Positioning of the patient

- Safety of patient
- Skin preparation
- Draping routine
- Assisting of physician or anesthesiologist
- Transport of patient to postprocedure area
- Preparation of suite for next procedural case
- Radiation safety

Postprocedural Routine

- Monitor final vital signs before transfer
- Report to postoperative care nurse and transfer patient
- Document transfer in record
- Maintain patient safety

Employment Application

Name: _____   Date: _____

Address: _____   How long at this address? _____

City, State, and ZIP: _____

Home Telephone: _____   Cell Phone: _____

E-mail Address: _____   Social Security No.: _____

Prior Addresses for the Last Five Years (list in reverse order)	Dates of Residence (mm/yy)	
	From	To

EMPLOYMENT EXPERIENCE

Start with your present job or last job. Include military assignments and other volunteer activities. Exclude organizational names that indicate race, color, religion, sex, or national origin. We may contact the employers you list unless you inform us otherwise and provide a reason.

Employer 1 _____

Address _____ City _____ State _____ Zip _____

Telephone No. _____ Supervisor's Name _____

Job Title _____ Reason for Leaving _____

Dates of Employment: From _____ To _____   Salary or Hourly Rate _____

Employer 2 _____

Address _____ City _____ State _____ Zip _____

Telephone No. _____ Supervisor's Name _____

Job Title _____ Reason for Leaving _____

Dates of Employment: From _____ To _____   Salary or Hourly Rate _____

Employer 3 _____

Address _____ City _____ State _____ Zip _____

Telephone No. _____ Supervisor's Name _____

Job Title _____ Reason for Leaving _____

Dates of Employment: From _____ To _____   Salary or Hourly Rate _____

EDUCATION

	Name and Location	No. of Years Attended	Graduation Year	Degree
High School				
College				
Graduate				
Other				

OTHER SPECIAL TRAINING OR SKILLS YOU POSSESS OR LANGUAGES YOU SPEAK AND/OR WRITE

_____

_____

_____

_____

Driver's License No.: _____   State: _____   Expiration: _____

Are you a veteran of the US military service?   ☐ Yes ☐ No

Are you a citizen of the United States of America?   ☐ Yes ☐ No

Do you have the legal right to permanently work in the United States?   ☐ Yes ☐ No

Have you ever been convicted of a crime?   ☐ Yes ☐ No

Have you applied here before?   ☐ Yes ☐ No

When are you available to start work? _____

Are there any limitations on your travel or transfer to another office location? ☐ Yes ☐ No

What are your approximate salary requirements? _____

OFFICE SKILLS

_____

_____

_____

_____

REFERENCES

Name	Occupation	Address	Telephone Number

By signing this application, I certify that this application is complete and accurate to the best of my knowledge and that I have not made any attempt to conceal information and that falsification could be cause for dismissal. Furthermore, [insert practice name] or its agents may request employment information from my previous employers and persons or corporations who provide information related to my previous employment and will be released from any liability or damage. I understand this application is not intended to be a contract of employment. I have noted that [insert practice name] is an Equal Opportunity Employer and that ad applicants receive lawful consideration for employment without regard to race, religion, color, sex, age, national origin, disability, veteran status, marital status, or in the presence of a nonrelated medical condition or handicap. I realize that if I am hired, [insert practice name] reserves the right to terminate my employment whenever the need arises.

_____   _____
Signature   Date

Individual Employee Education Record

Instructions: Employees are responsible for keeping this education record current. All educational requirements must be met in order to be considered for your annual increase. Using this record, maintain a current list of all educational requirements completed during the calendar year.

Employee Name:	
DOH:	Position:

Certifications	
Type	**Expiration Date**

Staff Meeting Attendance					
Month	**Initial Attendance**	**Minutes Read**	**Month**	**Initial Attendance**	**Minutes Read**
January			July		
February			August		
March			September		
April			October		
May			November		
June			December		

Class/In-service/Module	Date Completed	Signature
Requirements must be completed annually.		
Workplace Violence		
Sexual Harassment		
Employee Health		
Safety OSHA		
Mandatory Education: In-services, Modules, Classes		

Applicant: _____   Date: _____

Interviewer: _____

Why did you apply for this job?
_____

If you could design the ideal job for yourself, what would it be like?
_____

Why did you leave your last job?
_____

What did you like best about your last job?
_____

What did you like least about your last job?
_____

May I contact your present employer as one of your references?
_____

What characteristics about yourself do you like best?
_____

Tell me about your qualifications and skills for this position.
_____

What motivates you to do an outstanding job?
_____

Describe a project, change, or procedure you designed or helped to implement that (1) helped serve patients better, (2) saved money, or (3) made money for your previous employer.
_____

What are some of the problems you have encountered in working with supervisors, colleagues, and patients? How did you handle them?
_____

How flexible can you be in your workdays and hours?
_____

Describe your short- and long-term career goals.
_____

What accomplishments or projects are you most proud of?
_____

Evaluation Key: 4 = excellent, 3 = good, 2 = satisfactory, 1 = poor			
	On time for appointment		Personal appearance
	Conducts self professionally		Discreet/confidential
	Speaks clearly		Hygiene
	Pleasing personality		Open to learning
	Cheerful, interested		Self-confident
	Seems truthful		Listens

Information and Forms for New Employees

Check if Completed	Information and Forms	Supervisor's Signature	Employee's Signature
☐	Time card	_____	_____
☐	Insurance forms and information	_____	_____
☐	W-2 form	_____	_____
☐	I-9 form	_____	_____
☐	Policy and procedure manual	_____	_____
☐	Job description	_____	_____
☐	Name tag	_____	_____
☐	Key control log	_____	_____

Note: All information listed above must be signed off by the employee and supervisor.

Payroll Service Outsourcing

If you are thinking of using an outside payroll service, the following points are a few things you should know as you find a firm and solicit 3 bids.

Notes

☐   It can take one employee up to 2 hours per pay period to do all the payroll tasks for a staff or 5 or 6. More staff would require more time.   _____

☐   Could this employee use this time on a more profitable task such as billing or collections?   _____

☐   It may be more cost effective to have the following tasks provided by a payroll service: _____

- o   Calculating and recording payroll taxes

- o   Writing checks

- o   Mailing checks

- o   Handling direct deposits

- o   Providing information for tax forms (corporate forms)

- o   Providing W-2 and W-3 forms

- o   Paying payroll taxes

- o   Preparing 941 and 940 forms

Personnel File

Employee Name	Position/Title	Date of Hire	Application	Job Description Signed Y/N	Orientation Skills Checklist	License Verification	License Expiration Date	Health Questionnaire	PPD Testing Date Due	OSHA/BHW Training	Risk Management Initial Training	Risk Management Annual Training	BCLS Expiration Date	ACLS (if applicable) Expiration Date	Hepatitis B Vaccine Documentation	90-Day Evaluation Due	Annual Evaluation Due	Reference Check Done	Confidentiality Statement on File

[electronic file name and path]

Created: [Date]

Personnel Records Maintenance List

Notes

☐ You must retain all of your ex-employees' records for 7 years or longer. _____

☐ Retain all job applications and resumes for at least 2 years, even for those not hired. _____

Retain the following payroll records for each employee to guarantee that your practice is meeting Fair Labor Standard Act (FLSA) requirements.

☐ Job title _____

☐ Date of birth if younger than 19 years _____

☐ Home address, including ZIP code _____

☐ Sex _____

☐ Full name as used in Social Security records _____

☐ Earnings for salaried (straight-time) employees, wages, and overtime due _____

☐ Total wages paid each pay period _____

☐ Date of each paycheck and the pay period it covers _____

☐ The hours worked each day and week in each pay period _____

☐ Day and time of the week on which employee's workweek begins _____

☐ All pay information for each pay period. This includes dates, amounts of increase or decrease with description. _____

Recruitment: Marketing Applicants to Become Patients

		Responsible Party	Notes
1	Your classified ad for job openings should be positive and attention grabbing.	_____	_____
2	When writing your ad, you want the practice to be attractive to future applicants and patients.	_____	_____
3	Display your practice name prominently in your ads and any advertising and letterhead.	_____	_____
4	Have a packet of information on your practice to give to each applicant after the interview or by mail for those not interviewed.	_____	_____
5	If you have a newsletter, you can mail a complimentary copy to all applicants.	_____	_____
6	Give all applicants a short tour of your facility; this may bring them back as patients even if they are not hired.	_____	_____
7	After the interview process, sending a small thank you gift leaves a good impression, and the person may be more inclined to mention your practice to friends and family.	_____	_____
8	Add the names of rejected applicants to your mailing list. You can send them invitations to future open houses, etc.	_____	_____

Time Sheet

	Pay Period No.
Name	**Employee No.**

Time	Sun	Mon	Tue	Wed	Thu	Fri	Sat
Start							
Lunch Break: In/Out							
Stop							
O/T							
TOTAL							

Absences During Time Period

	Available	Used
Sick Leave		
Personal		
Vacation		

_____   _____
Employee's Signature   Date

_____   _____
Employer's Signature   Date

Manager Training on Employee Confidentiality

Check if Completed		Responsible Party	Notes
☐	Never counsel an employee in front of co-workers.	_____	_____
☐	Do not put irrelevant information in personnel files.	_____	_____
☐	Discourage gossip by not partaking in it yourself.	_____	_____
☐	Do not talk to employees about other employees. Personal information is available only to other personnel on a "need to know" basis.	_____	_____
☐	When collecting personal information from your employees, let them know what you need it for.	_____	_____
☐	Do not discuss the reasons for an employee's absence.	_____	_____
☐	Employees have the right to inspect their personnel files.	_____	_____
☐	Employees who are also patients must sign all patient privacy forms.	_____	_____
☐	Do not release the contents of personnel files to anyone without the employee's knowledge or a court order.	_____	_____

New Employee Personnel Training

Check if Completed		Responsible Party	Notes
☐	Determine staffing needs	_____	_____
☐	Check local resources for personnel	_____	_____
☐	Determine whether anyone currently employed is a good candidate	_____	_____
☐	Start interviewing for office/clinical personnel as soon as position is available	_____	_____

Review Practice Guidelines on Patient Appointment Scheduling Methods and Preferences

☐	Staff meeting and communications effectiveness	_____	_____
☐	Telephone techniques	_____	_____
☐	OSHA bloodborne pathogens policy	_____	_____
☐	HIPAA compliance policy	_____	_____
☐	Personnel policies	_____	_____
☐	Determine appropriate amount and type of slot on the basis of schedule matrix (Tool 03003)	_____	_____
☐	Check patient's account; if delinquent, arrange for payment upon patient's arrival.	_____	_____

Review Checking Patients In Protocols

☐	Have patient sign in.	_____	_____
☐	Copy front and back of insurance card, even if an established patient	_____	_____
☐	Patient data collection sheets; have patient update outdated information	_____	_____
☐	Handling a delinquent account	_____	_____
☐	Encounter tickets—why serially numbered	_____	_____
☐	Review route of encounter form	_____	_____

Checkout: Receptionist

Check if Completed		Responsible Party	Notes
☐	Adjustment policy: who can make adjustments?	_____	_____
☐	Collection of copayment and deductible	_____	_____
☐	Financial Policy: verify current ICD-9-CM and CPT codebooks on hand (physician key in accurate coding; coding CPE critically important for physician and staff)	_____	_____

Billing and Reimbursement Protocols

☐	Participant or Non-Participant status with Medicare?	_____	_____
☐	Collections procedures and collections letters	_____	_____
☐	Adjustment policy: who can make adjustments?	_____	_____
☐	Why physician approval of each initial daysheet	_____	_____

Manager Training on Successful Interviews and Recruitment

Notes

☐   Job applicants will judge you on how well you know them from the application and resume. Read application well before the interview begins.

_____   _____

☐   Explain duties for the job that they have applied for.

_____   _____

☐   Neat and professional appearance sets the standard for employees to follow.

_____   _____

☐   Do not tell applicants they will hear from you if you do not intend to hire them. They also prefer a telephone call as opposed to a letter.

_____   _____

☐   Keep the questions related to the job being interviewed for.

_____   _____

☐   Do not sell the job to make it sound too good to be true. You do not want the applicant leaving with any suspicious thoughts. Thoroughly explain the position's strengths and weaknesses.

_____   _____

☐   Introduce applicants to current employees.

_____   _____

Drug Screening Through Urinalysis
Applicant Consent

I, _____, understand that as part of the
(print applicant's full name)

pre-employment process [practice] may conduct a comprehensive background investigation for the purpose of

determining my suitability to fill the position for which I have applied. I further understand that I will be required to

submit to a drug-screening test prior to the offer of employment. This is all in accordance with the policy of

[practice] to maintain a workforce that is free of illegal drug and alcohol abuse. In accordance with this policy, I

consent to have an appropriate specimen collected and tested for any and all controlled substances.

I do hereby voluntarily consent to the sampling and submission for testing of my urine for the purpose of screening

for the presence of illegal drugs and/or an abusive level of prescribed medication. I understand that a negative

result from this screening is a condition of employment.

I also understand that producing a positively confirmed test result for the presence of illegal drugs and/or an

abusive level of prescribed medication will result in the rejection of my application for employment. I understand

that a confirmed positive test result indicating the presence of illegal drugs and/or an abusive level of prescribed

medication will bar me from securing employment with [practice] for at least one year.

_____

Name of Applicant (including maiden name)—please print

_____

Signature of Applicant

_____

Social Security Number

_____

Date

Leave Request

Date Request Made:		
Employee Name:		Employee Number:
Requested Day(s) Off:		
Reason for Request:		

Deduct as: ❑ Vacation/Sick Leave   ❑ Compensation Time   ❑ From Payroll

❑ Approved	❑ Not Approved	Initials:		Date:	
Comments:					

❑ Approved	❑ Not Approved	Initials:		Date:	
Comments:					

❑ Approved	❑ Not Approved	Initials:		Date:	
Comments:					

Record of Keys Issued

Name	Date Issued	Type of Key

Request for Expense Reimbursement

Please complete the following information for any expense for which you are requesting reimbursement.

Name: _____   Date of request: _____

Purpose of expenditures: _____

List of expenses requested: _____

Date	Expense Paid To Whom	Amount
	Travel: Auto-private (_____¢ per mile)	
	TOTAL	

If your expenses are for a meeting, please make sure to list the cost of meals and the registration for the meeting separately.

All requests for reimbursement must have receipts attached to the request for verification.

Mileage (private auto) is payable at the present rate on the date which the expense occurred.

Approved by: _____   Date: _____

Copyright ©2009 American Medical Association

Tuition Assistance

Employee Name: _____

Employee Number: _____

Course Name	Credit Hours	Grade	School

Comments (Note cost here):

_____

❑ Approved   ❑ Disapproved

_____   _____

Supervisor's Signature   Date

(Attach copies of receipts for tuition cost to this form.)

Notice of Injury by Industrial Accident

Date: _____

To: _____ (Manager or Supervisor)

Please take notice that I was injured by industrial accident on [date] by [describe briefly how the accident happened].

Type of injury: _____

Witnesses (if any): _____

Physicians seen, if any: _____

Hospital or emergency department treatment, if any: _____

This accident should be reported to the Workers' Compensation Commission, as required by law, and acknowledgment of this notice should be given to the employee.

Signature: _____

(Note: The employee must complete a First Report of Injury.)

Workers' Compensation Form for Treatment

Company:	

Contact Person:		Insurer:	
Telephone No.:		Policy No.:	
Address:		Telephone No.:	

Approval of Service	Special Billing Instructions
1. Employee must have authorization form (pink) with him or her, or call before treatment	1. First report must be sent directly to [insert information]
2. Obtain employee ID badge before treatment	2. Treatment plan to be sent to [insert information] with billing form (CMS-1500).

Special Report Requirements

1. Copy first report and send to [insert information]
2. Treatment plan and possible date of work return form to be completed within five days of first treatment.

Date of update: ____/____/____

By: _____

Occupational Health Information Card
Note: Use a 5 x 8 index card and file alphabetically by employer (company)

chapter | 11

Human Resources

Performance appraisal is often an unpopular topic; however, when appraisals are based on clear, fair expectations, they can provide the basis for the betterment of individual employees and of the practice. Expectations of employees are stated in job descriptions and policies and procedures. They should be clear, the same for employees in similar positions with similar experience, and clearly related to the job. When expectations meet these criteria, developing a performance appraisal tool and conducting the appraisal become less daunting. In addition, in a work environment that fosters inquiry; cooperation; inclusion of employees in decision making; equality among patients, physicians, and supervisory, clinical, clerical, and technical staff; and blame-free problem identification and resolution, performance appraisal can be viewed as an opportunity for growth rather than a necessary evil.

As the number of employees grows in a practice, consideration needs to be given to the focus of supervisory personnel. Modern-day supervision involves much more than making sure employees arrive on time and perform their assignments, so supervisors need sufficient time for their supervisory duties. When supervisors assess employee performance, they need to consider all aspects of the performance, including the effects of the systems and processes in the practice on the performance of an individual or a group of employees. Analyzing problems and identifying root causes could take a substantial amount of a supervisor's time, but the time pays off because future problems can be reduced or prevented.

Employee compensation involves not only money, but also scheduling, benefits, and paid time off. Compensation needs to be competitive with that of other practices in the area to attract and retain quality employees. A practice needs to determine which benefits will be provided, such as health insurance and day care, and to develop policies on holidays, vacation time accrual, and sick leave and family leave. Employees who are well compensated, given work schedules that provide time to manage their personal lives, and included in decisions that affect patient care processes and their work lives are likely to be loyal, hard working, and productive. Periodic review of compensation packages should be done by comparing practice policies against peer practices or medical group management associations, or by contacting a certified health care business consultant (https://www.nschbc.org).

The tools in this chapter are designed to assist practices in developing wage scales, appraisal tools, and personnel policies. In addition, Tool 02001 in Chapter 2 provides a form for evaluation of an associate physician, a physician assistant, or a nurse practitioner.

Staff development encompasses orientation to the practice and the specific position, ongoing training as changes are instituted or problems are identified, and further personal and professional development. A staff development program provides opportunities to enrich and enhance personnel and is an essential part of recruitment and retention of qualified staff.

Increasing their knowledge and skill empowers employees and makes the practice more productive. Empowered employees are able to initiate problem identification and resolution and participate in analysis that leads to identification of root causes and solutions likely to work. But, because management has so often been from the top down, employees often need to know how to handle empowerment. Staff development can teach employees how to identify and communicate problems and concerns and how to participate in resolution. It can also influence the ability of employees to collaborate with staff in their own and other departments, staff at other agencies, and, primarily, patients. The checklists in this chapter are designed to help staff in selected areas.

Tools for Human Resources

Number	Title	Purpose	Notes
11001	Form for Establishing a Compensation Scale	To provide guidance in establishing pay grades	Grades are established according to the importance of the job to the practice. Steps within the grades recognize experience, length of service to the practice, and competence. Theoretically, the salary at the highest step within a grade is near the entry salary for the next highest grade. This tool includes two forms. One tool bases salaries on years of service and the type of position. The other divides each grade into quartiles, or steps.
11002	Form for Creating a Total Compensation Statement	To provide employees with information about their total compensation and the cost associated with their employment	
11003	Form for Counseling	To document counseling	Documentation data for counseling sessions can be used to track improvement and whether the action to resolve the problem was effective. These data can also help identify whether the problem is related to a specific employee or to the systems and processes in place at the practice.
11004	Form for an Employee Complaint	To provide employees with a means to file a written complaint	Data related to employee complaints can be used in the same ways as the data in Tool 11003.

Number	Title	Purpose	Notes
11005	Form for Employee Progressive Conduct Offenses	To provide a format for managing employee conduct offenses	
11006	Form for Employee Corrective Action	To document a problem situation, corrective action, and the employee's response	
11007	Form for Patient or Employee Incident and Action Taken	To report an employee incident and the action to be taken	The information obtained and the action plan are designed for nonpunitive identification and correction of problems.
11008	Form for an Introductory Employee Evaluation	To review the performance of an employee during the probationary period	
11009	Form for a Clinical Employee Performance Review	To review an employee's performance	This form is for the evaluation of a laboratory employee.
11010	Form for Administrative Employee Performance Review	To review an employee's performance	This form is for reviewing administrative employees.
11011	Form for an Employee Termination/Exit Interview	To document an exit interview	Data on this form can be used to determine whether a problem exists that needs to addressed by the practice.
11012	Form for an Employee Wage/Salary History	To track of an employee's salary	
11013	Form for Manager Self-Assessment	To provide a tool for self-assessment of a manager's supervisory skills	
11014	Form for a Performance Review	To review employee performance	
11015	Template for Investigating and Responding to Claims of Harassment and Discrimination	To identify steps for dealing with harassment and discrimination in the workplace	
11016	Checklist for Motivating Employees	To identify ways to motivate employees	

Number	Title	Purpose	Notes
11017	Checklist for a Issuing a Directive	To identify strategies for issuing a directive, when necessary	Few people like being told what to do, but sometimes a directive is necessary.
11018	Checklist for Holiday Incentives	To identify ideas for holiday gifts and incentives	

Years of Service	Nurse	Medical Technician	Receptionist
10			
9			
8			
7			
6			
5			
4			
3			
2			
1			

Grade	1st	2nd	3rd	4th
A				
B				
C				
D				
E				
F				
G				

Total Compensation Statement

Employee Name:_____

Calendar Year Ending:_____

We want you to know the total compensation (salary and benefits) that [practice name] was pleased to provide for you during the calendar year [insert year].

Wages/Salary	$_____
Bonuses	$_____
Social Security Payroll Taxes	$_____
Unemployment Payroll Taxes	$_____
Health Insurance/Medical Reimbursement	$_____
Dental Services	$_____
Continuing Education	$_____
Pension/Retirement Plan	$_____
Uniform Allowance	$_____
Professional Dues	$_____
Other	$_____
Other	$_____
Total Compensation and Benefits for [insert year]	$_____
Total Hours Worked in [insert year]	$_____
Total Compensation and Benefits per Hour in [insert year]	$_____

We are happy that these compensation and benefits could be provided for you and hope that the next year will be even better. Thank you for your service.

Mandatory Annual Training Control Log

Name	Position	Type of Training Control (CPR, OSHA, CLIA, Domestic Violence, or HIPAA)	Certification No. (if required)	Training Date

Date: _____

Please describe the problem/conflict. _____

_____

_____

_____

_____

What is the history of the problem? _____

_____

_____

_____

_____

What action has been taken on your complaint? _____

_____

_____

_____

What action do you feel should be taken? _____

_____

_____

_____

_____

Additional comments: _____

_____

_____

Employee's Name: _____

Supervisor: _____

Date of meeting with Office Manager: _____

Resolved: ☐ Yes   ☐ No

Action taken by office: _____

_____

_____

_____

_____

Employee Conduct Offenses

Group One Offenses

First offense: Verbal consultation
Second offense: Written conference
Third offense: Three-day suspension without pay
Fourth offense: Discharge

- Behavior that is disruptive to other employees, patients, or [insert name of practice] operations
- Excessive time spent on breaks, lunch, or away from your designated work area
- Disregard for [insert name of practice]'s established dress codes
- Excessive personal telephone calls, incoming (cell phones included) or telephone calls placed during working hours. (Cell telephones should be on the vibrate mode, except those cell phones that are receiving business-related telephone calls.)
- Negligence in observing fire prevention and established safety rules or regulations
- Leaving work without permission during normal work shift or leaving work early without prior authorization
- Conducting personal work on paid time
- Committing, allowing, or contributing to unsanitary, unsafe, or disorderly conditions at work
- Failure to meet job performance standards relating to the quality, quantity, or timeliness of work while in a nonprobationary status
- Removal or altering of any posted materials
- Failure to report for a mandatory meeting and/or failure to report in a timely manner

Group Two Offenses

First offense: Written conference
Second offense: Five-day suspension without pay
Third offense: Discharge

- Inability to meet expectations of job performance relating to accuracy of charts, lab results, patient information, etc, that ultimately affect the patient and/or practice
- Using profane language during working hours
- Insubordinate behavior or refusal to comply with instructions or failure to perform reasonable duties, which are properly assigned
- Unauthorized use of practice material, time, equipment, or property
- Sexual harassment
- Throwing things, horseplay, practical jokes, disorderly conduct, or any other display of workplace violence, which may endanger or interrupt the well-being of any employee, patient, or visitor on practice premises
- Soliciting gifts or gratuities from patients, visitors, vendors, staff, or physicians
- Discourteous treatment of patients, visitors, or other employees
- Failure to comply with [insert name of practice]'s no smoking policy
- Failure to follow appropriate guidelines for calling in sick or absent

Group Three Offenses

First offense: Five-day suspension without pay
Second offense: Discharge

- Discussion between employees of employee's rates of pay
- Unauthorized possession of practice or employee property, gambling, or violating criminal laws on company premises
- Threatening, intimidating, coercing, or interfering with the performance of other employees
- Excessive tardiness or absenteeism
- Conduct outside [insert name of practice] that the practice feels reflects adversely on the employee or practice
- Damaging or destroying practice property as a result of careless or willful acts
- Theft of practice property or that of a fellow employee, patient, physician, or visitor
- Poor performance in any aspect of the job that, in the practice's opinion, does not meet the requirements of the position
- Administration of medication without a license or in violation of other applicable laws, statutes, or [insert name of practice] policy

- Unauthorized use or release of confidential information, including discussing confidential information with individuals not associated with [insert name of practice]

Group Four Offenses

First offense: Discharge

- Possession, consumption, or distribution of illegal drugs, alcohol, narcotics, or unauthorized substances while on [insert name of practice] premises or while on practice time
- Reporting to work or working with impaired abilities
- Fighting or assault with a dangerous weapon
- Possession of a firearm, explosives, or any other dangerous or illegal weapon while on [insert name of practice] premises
- Falsifying any [insert name of practice] records or documents
- Falsifying employment application or any information obtained during the interview process
- Conduct that violates common decency or moral values
- Deliberately falsifying or altering your time sheet/time card or that of any individual other than yourself
- Deliberate destruction of patient, employee, physician, or [insert name of practice] property
- Violation of any civil rights prohibited by law
- Threatening to or rendering physical harm to patients, employees, physicians, or visitors
- Engaging in such other practices as the practice determines may be inconsistent with the ordinary and reasonable rules of conduct necessary to the welfare of the practice, its employees, or patients, including acts of dishonesty, fraud, theft, sabotage, conviction, or imprisonment

Corrective Action Form

Employee Name: _____ Job Title: _____

1. Type of Action: ☐ Verbal Consultation ☐ Written Conference ☐ Suspension ☐ Discharge

2. Describe the situation that occurred; be specific in stating observable behaviors, performance and policy violations. Please include date(s), time(s), other employees involved, other people involved, and any other pertinent contributing circumstances or factors.

_____

_____

_____

_____

_____

_____

_____

_____

3. Effect this situation had on employee's work, other employees, or the practice.

_____

_____

_____

_____

_____

_____

_____

_____

_____

_____ _____
Supervisor's Signature   Date

_____ _____
Physician's Signature   Date

4.   Specifically what actions are to be accomplished by the employee to improve?

_____

_____

_____

_____

_____

_____

_____

5.   Reassessment follow-up date: _____

6.   Consequences of failing to meet performance expectations by follow-up review date:

_____

_____

_____

_____

_____

_____

_____

_____

_____

_____

☐   My supervisor has reviewed the above situation with me and the attached sheet has my following comments.

☐   I agree with this review and have no additional comments and/or information that I wish to document.

☐   I have received a copy of this form as well as any other attached sheets. I understand that if I disagree with this disciplinary action, I am encouraged to speak with the Employee Relations Manager.

_____   _____

Employee's Signature   Date

Corrective Action Form
Additional Employee Comments

_____

_____

_____

_____

_____

_____

_____

_____

_____

_____

_____

_____

_____

_____

_____

_____

_____

_____

_____

_____

_____

_____

_____

_____

_____

_____

_____   _____

Employee's Signature   Date

Incident Management Investigation Report

Report of Investigation Findings: What Did the True Cause Investigation and Analysis Find?

What factors are involved in the event (eg, human, equipment, controllable environment, uncontrollable external factors)?

_____

_____

_____

What systems or processes underlie these factors (eg, human resources issues, information management issues, emergency and failure-mode responses, leadership issues, uncontrollable factors)?

_____

_____

_____

Patient Outcomes:

_____

_____

_____

Corrective Action to Be Taken as a Result of Investigation Findings

What will you do to prevent reoccurrence of the incident?

_____

_____

_____

Action Plan

True Cause/ Opportunity for Improvement	Action to Reduce Reoccurrence	Persons(s) Responsible for Implementation	Date of Implementation	Result Expected

Person Responsible for Reviewing the Findings: _____

Date of Review of Report: _____

Person Responsible for Communicating Findings to Employee: _____

Date of Communications Report: _____

Follow-up Actions to Be Taken (check all appropriate actions)

☐   No action required

☐   Communication of findings to staff

☐   Staff training and in-service

☐   Development of new policy/procedure

☐   Revision of policy/procedure

☐   Staff competency assessment

☐   Cease patient testing

☐   Refer patient testing

☐   Resume patient testing

☐   Other

Corrective Action Monitoring

☐   Corrective action follow-up and review by following date:_____

☐   Findings inconclusive; monitor process and review by following date:_____

☐   Information incomplete; follow-up to be completed by following date: _____

Report Submitted By: _____   Date: _____

Report Approved By: _____   Date: _____

Facility Information (complete all information)

Facility Name: _____   Laboratory: _____

Director: _____   Date: _____

Address: _____   Telephone: _____

_____   Fax No.: _____

City, State: _____   ZIP Code: _____

Person Reporting Event: _____   Date: _____

Reporting Information (complete all information)

| **Date of Incident** | **Number of Persons Affected** |

Incident: _____   Patient(s): _____

_____   Staff: _____

Time: _____   Other(s): _____

Event Type (check all appropriate event types)

☐ Death related to treatment   ☐ Death related to medication error based on lab result

☐ Injury due to treatment   ☐ Failure in safety procedure

☐ Misidentification of specimen   ☐ Hemolytic blood transfusion reaction

☐ Misidentification of report   ☐ Procedures involving the wrong patient

☐ Misdiagnosis based on laboratory report   ☐ Procedures involving the wrong body part

☐ Instruments or materials retained in the   ☐ Recurring complaints about phlebotomy or specimen
   patient following a procedure   collection

☐ Physical attack or abduction   ☐ Instrument and methodology failures

☐ Other catastrophic event (describe): _____

Patient/Staff Information of Person Affected by Event (complete all Information)

Name (last, first, middle): _____   _____   _____

Date of Birth: _____   Patient Identification Number: _____

Current Status: ☐ Discharged   ☐ Hospitalized   ☐ Deceased   ☐ Unknown

Treatment Date: _____

Person Responsible for Investigation of Event: _____

Date of Investigation Report: _____

Regulatory Agency to be Notified of Incident: _____

Date of Notification: _____

Ordering Physician to be Notified of Incident: _____

Date of Notification: _____

Person to be Notified of Incident: _____

Date of Notification: _____

Brief Summary of Incident

What happened, and how was it handled? What area is affected?

_____

_____

_____

_____

_____

_____

_____

_____

_____

_____

_____

_____

_____

Important: Please return this form by _____ .

Employee Name _____   Employee Number _____   Date _____

Position _____   Department _____   Date employed _____

SUPERVISOR'S RATING

Evaluate and rate each of the qualities listed.	Satisfactory	Unsatisfactory	Unable to Rate	Comments
Attendance				
Punctuality				
Personal appearance and habits				
Learning rate				
Quality of work				
Quantity of work				
Suitability for position				

In comparison with employees performing similar job functions and with the same length of service, how would you rate this employee?

☐ Outstanding   ☐ Above average   ☐ Average   ☐ Fair   ☐ Unsatisfactory

SUPERVISOR'S RECOMMENDATION

Do you recommend that this employee be retained as a regular employee?   ☐ Yes   ☐ No

If no, please specify the reasons why he/she should not be retained. Provides as much detail as possible.

_____

_____

_____

_____

_____

_____

Employee Name: _____   **Employee Number:** _____

Job Title: _____

Skills	Outstanding	Good	Satisfactory	Poor
Venipuncture				
Laboratory testing				
Interviewing patients				
Reporting test results				
Communication with physicians				
Communication with management				
Peer relationships				

Note: The skills and other aspects that are evaluated will vary for each person. Also, the employee is encouraged to evaluate himself or herself using this form prior to performance review

Comments: _____

_____

_____

Employee Salary: _____ as of _____

Recommended Salary Increase (if applicable): _____

Effective Date of Increase: _____

_____   _____
Employee's Signature   Date

_____   _____
Supervisor's Signature   Date

Employee Name: _____   Employee Number: _____

Job Title: _____

Skills	Outstanding	Good	Satisfactory	Poor
Telephone technique				
Scheduling appointments				
Communication with patients				
Accuracy of data input				
Collection of copayments and deductibles				
Communication with physicians				
Communication with management				
Peer relationships				

Note: The skills and other aspects that are evaluated will vary for each person. Also, the employee is encouraged to evaluate himself or herself using this form prior to performance review

Comments: _____

_____

_____

Employee Salary: _____ as of _____

Recommended Salary Increase (if applicable): _____

Effective Date of Increase: _____

_____   _____
Employee's Signature   Date

_____   _____
Supervisor's Signature   Date

_____   _____
Employee Name   Date

_____   _____
Date of Termination   Last Day of Work

_____   _____
Name of Exit Interviewer   Date

Note to the employee: All comments will be maintained confidential.

Have all keys and/or other employer property been returned?   ☐ Yes   ☐ No

Has the employee been given all information regarding the following?

Insurance coverage   ☐ Yes   ☐ No
Benefits coverage and limitation   ☐ Yes   ☐ No
Final pay   ☐ Yes   ☐ No

What is the reason for leaving?   _____

_____

_____

Is the employee aware of any issues regarding the employer that need to be handled, including but not limited to, the following?

Billing issues   ☐ Yes   ☐ No
Employee problems   ☐ Yes   ☐ No
Security Issues   ☐ Yes   ☐ No
Breaches of stated policies   ☐ Yes   ☐ No

If yes, explain.   _____

_____

_____

Other suggestions: _____

_____

_____

_____   _____
Employee Signature   Date

Health Benefits Expire: _____

References to be given by: _____

_____

Nature of Reference: _____

Rehire?   ☐ Yes   ☐ No

Confidential Employee Wage/Salary History

Employee Name: _____   Employee Number: _____

Dates		Position and Classification	Work Location	Rate of Pay		Reason for Change
From	To			Amount	Per	

Created: [Date]

Manager Self-Assessment Quiz

Self-Assessment Objectives	Meet objective always	Meet objectives most times	Meet objective sometimes	Do not meet objectives
Maintain productivity of my employees	4	3	2	0
Delegate authority	4	3	2	0
Encourage all employees	4	3	2	0
Treat employees fairly	4	3	2	0
Focus on how to correct an employee's mistake, rather than blaming the employee	4	3	2	0
Give employees specific ways to improve performance	4	3	2	0
Keep all employee counseling private	4	3	2	0
Demonstrate that I am approachable	4	3	2	0
Notice and praise employees who show improvement	4	3	2	0
Explain reasons for the tasks I assign	4	3	2	0
When giving instructions, give all the information necessary to perform it well	4	3	2	0
Ask, rather than order, employees to perform a tasks, if possible	4	3	2	0
Total points for each column				=

Total Score _____

48 points: You are an excellent supervisor.

36–47 points: You manage effectively but need improvement.

22-35 points: You're moderately effective, and some of your management skills could be sharpened.

21 or less points: Your management skills need to be improved before the next evaluation process.

Overall Subjective Performance Review

Employee: _____

Reviewer: _____

Date: _____

	Excellent	Satisfactory	Needs Improvement	Unacceptable
Accepts and follows established rules and procedures				
Accepts changes in routine and procedures				
Communicates openly orally and in writing				
Completes work on time				
Conducts self in a professional manner with patients				
Cooperates and works well with people				
Demonstrates good attendance and punctuality				
Does share of workload				
Has an interest in job and patients				
Leaves personal affairs at home				
Makes efficient use of time				
Notices what needs to be done and does it without being told				
Organizes work efficiently and practically				
Performs well under pressure				
Performs with minimal supervision				
Maintains professional personal appearance				
Provides patient education				
Puts original and constructive thinking into practice				
Respects confidential information, both patient and personal				

	Excellent	Satisfactory	Needs Improvement	Unacceptable
Employee: _____				
Reviewer: _____				
Date: _____				
Respects other person's opinion even if in disagreement				
Responds to directions quickly				
Seeks new knowledge and skills				
Takes care of own health				
Uses language becoming a professional				
Work is neat and legible				
[Insert additional performance criteria]				
[Insert additional performance criteria]				
[Insert additional performance criteria]				
[Insert additional performance criteria]				
[Insert additional performance criteria]				

I have discussed this review with the employee.

_____   _____

Reviewer's Signature   *Date*

I have read and understand this review and received a copy of it.

_____   _____

Employee's Signature   *Date*

Investigating and Responding to Claims of Harassment and Discrimination

NOTE: Always contact the administrator before conducting an investigation.

I. **Thoroughly investigate the complaint immediately.**
   A. Investigate *every* complaint.
      1. Failure to investigate the claim may be seen as "tacit approval" of the harasser's activities.
      2. Thorough investigations will help insulate the employer from a harasser's potential claims that his or her discharge or discipline was unlawful.
   B. Keep the investigation and the facts that it uncovers under a strict "need to know" basis.
   C. Interview the complainant, the accused, the accused's supervisor, and witnesses as soon as possible. Take written statements.

II. **Step 1: Interview the complainant**
   A. Remain objective. Ask objective questions
   B. Determine the identity of the accused harasser(s).
   C. Determine when and where the incident occurred.
   D. Determine whether the incident was isolated or part of a series.
   E. Get specific details of the incident(s).
   F. Ask the complainant his or her reaction to the incident(s).
   G. Determine whether there were any witnesses to the incident(s).
   H. Determine whether the complainant has spoken to anyone else about the incident(s).
   I. Assure the complainant that the complaint will be taken seriously and investigated thoroughly.
   J. Assure the complainant that the complaint will be kept as confidential as possible, consistent with an appropriate investigation.
   K. Never agree to forgo an investigation of a complaint pursuant to the complainant's request for confidentiality.

III. **Step 2: Interview the accused**
   A. Remain objective. Ask objective questions.
   B. Determine whether the accused harasser knows of the incident or incidents to which the complainant is referring. If so:
      1. determine when and where the incident(s) took place;
      2. get specific details of the incident(s);
      3. ask how the complainant reacted;
      4. determine whether there were any witnesses to the incident(s); and
      5. determine whether the accused harasser has spoken to anyone else about the incident(s).
   C. Determine whether there was ever a prior consensual relationship between the parties.
   D. Determine the accused harasser's perception of his or her working relationship with the complainant.
   E. Ask whether the complainant and accused harasser socialized together alone or in a group.
   F. Determine whether the accused harasser(s) knows of any reason why the complainant would make the allegation.
   G. Determine whether the accused directed, or had responsibility for, the work of other employees or the complainant, had authority to recommend employment decisions affecting others, or was responsible for the maintenance or administration of the records of others.
   H. Observe the accused's demeanor and reaction.
   I. When the accused harasser is the complainant's supervisor, determine whether the complainant was recently granted or denied any job benefits, eg, raises, promotions.
   J. Assure the accused harasser that the complaint will be kept as confidential as possible, consistent with an appropriate investigation.

IV. **Step 3: Interview the accused's supervisor**
   A. Determine the accused's discipline problems or behavior patterns.
   B. Determine whether the supervisor had any knowledge about any relationship between the complainant and the accused.

C.   Determine whether the complainant ever reported the conduct to the supervisor.

V.   **Step 4: Interview witnesses when necessary**
   A.   Remain objective.
   B.   When the witness is a current or former employee, review his or her personnel file prior to the interview.
   C.   Inform the witness that the investigation is confidential. Inform current employees that a breach of confidentiality will result in disciplinary action.
   D.   Be alert to the privacy rights of the complainant and the accused harasser.
   E.   Do not give details of the complaint unless it is necessary to obtain relevant information.
   F.   Phrase questions so as not to give unnecessary information.
   G.   Do not automatically limit the investigation to witnesses currently in the workforce. Interview former employees, friends, and relatives of the complainant and the accused harasser if advised to do so by counsel.

VI.   **Step 5: Take corrective action**
   A.   Promptly take necessary corrective action, up to and including discharge. Corrective action must be effective. The employer's actions must guard against further harassing acts.
      1.   Consider the following: the severity of the conduct; the frequency; the pervasiveness of the conduct; whether you believe the individual will engage in further actions; and any past actions.
      2.   When imposing discipline on the harasser, any forms of discipline short of discharge should be given with a warning that similar misconduct in the future may result in immediate termination.
   B.   All corrective action taken must be documented. Include a summary of the investigation explaining the appropriateness of the action.

VII.   **Step 6: Follow through**
   A.   Inform the complainant that action was taken after thoroughly investigating the complaint.
   B.   Instruct the complainant to immediately report recurring or continuing harassment.
   C.   Show an interest in the complainant by periodically checking back with him or her to ensure that the harassment has been eliminated and is not continuing.

VIII.   **Step 7: Dealing with the accuser and the accused—Special situations**
   A.   The oversensitive accuser
      1.   Document and investigate the complaint as you would any other complaint.
      2.   If a reasonable person would not find the conduct abusive or offensive, nevertheless reassure the employee that the complaint was taken seriously. In most circumstances, the employer should not discipline or reprimand the accused.
      3.   If appropriate, explain the accuser's sensitivity to the accused and instruct the accused to stop the complained of conduct.
   B.   The accused committed nonsexual harassment.
      1.   Intimidation, hostility, name-calling or other types of abusive conduct directed toward others can be harassment.
      2.   In this situation, employers may have to remove individuals from the workplace if their mere presence would render the working environment hostile.
   C.   The accuser who informs a supervisor about harassing conduct, but wants to handle the problem himself or herself
      1.   The employer may be liable if it does not investigate and take corrective action because it has notice of harassing conduct in the workplace.
      2.   The supervisor should explain to the accuser that the company has a policy prohibiting harassment and that it has a duty to investigate the matter.
      3.   The supervisor should assure the accuser that the investigation will be conducted as confidentially as possible.
   D.   The company investigates a specific situation or anonymous complaints and rumors but cannot develop enough evidence to satisfy management that harassment occurred or to establish who is at fault.
      1.   To avoid future claims of inattention or tolerance of harassment, document to whom you spoke, what was said, etc. Conclude that the facts were inadequate to take individual action.
      2.   Consider using a memo or poster to all employees that reiterates the company's prohibition of harassment and the availability of the internal complaint procedure.
      3.   Ensure that managers and employees know the company is serious about taking disciplinary action under the policy.

Manger's Guide to Motivating Employees

Check if Completed		Responsible Party	Notes

Trust Building

☐ Give your employees opportunities to advance. _____ _____

☐ Reward successes. _____ _____

☐ Treat employees as partners, not peasants. _____ _____

Performance Appraisals Should Be Productive

☐ Have employees evaluate you. _____ _____

☐ Appraisals should not be routine; they should mean something and be helpful. _____ _____

☐ Goal setting should be a part of this process. _____ _____

☐ Set educational and performance goals. _____ _____

Develop Two-Way Communication

☐ Have an open-door policy; let staff know you really care. _____ _____

☐ Do not belittle employees for asking questions, even if the questions seem foolish. _____ _____

Personal Development for Your Employees

☐ Help employees set educational and personal goals. _____ _____

☐ Then ask what you can do to help staff members meet their goals. _____ _____

Empowering Employees in Decision Making

☐ Employees feel a part of the team; it can be very motivating when they are trusted to make some decisions. _____ _____

☐ Do not give employees more than they can responsibly handle. In other words, do not set them up to fail. _____ _____

Check if Completed		Responsible Party	Notes
	Delegating		
☐	Give the staff jobs with a higher level of responsibility, not just higher volume.	_____	_____
☐	The idea is to enrich the job, not enlarge it.	_____	_____
	Rewards		
☐	Do not be afraid to ask your employees what they would like to have.	_____	_____
☐	Sometimes cash is not always the best reward.	_____	_____

Issuing a Directive

☐   Thank the employee when appropriate.

☐   Follow up and provide feedback once the task has been performed.

☐   Make the directives plain and simple.

☐   Give step-by-step instructions if needed.

☐   Do not be condescending.

☐   Issue directives fairly and equally among staff.

☐   Do not leave any doubts as to who, where, when. and how it is to be done.

☐   Show the importance to those involved.

☐   Prepare employees so they are not surprised.

☐   Make sure you give the background and that the staff has the ability to meet the goal of the directive.

☐   Explain the need. Include facts and conditions that make it necessary.

☐   Limit the use of directives.

Holiday Incentive Ideas

Notes

☐   A visit from a consultant for a chair massage,   _____   _____
facial, or color makeover.

☐   Give a membership to a discount club,   _____   _____
travel club, spa, or gym.

☐   Close office and spend the afternoon at   _____   _____
a spa.

☐   Give subscriptions to popular magazines.   _____   _____

☐   Give your staff 4 hours off before the   _____   _____
holidays for some extra shopping time.

☐   Have a get-together where spouses   _____   _____
are invited as well. A party at your house
or a nice dinner out is always welcome.

☐   Make your last day before a holiday a half   _____   _____
day and take your staff out for a long lunch.

☐   Pay for a trip to a professional development   _____   _____
conference in a town that the employee
would like to visit.

☐   Personal enrichment classes at local   _____   _____
schools make nice gifts (eg, music lessons,
foreign language classes, cake decorating)

☐   Buy blocks of tickets for different games   _____   _____
and having the staff pick a game.

☐   Tickets to a night out on the town, a   _____   _____
dinner show, or theater tickets.

☐   Cash bonuses   _____   _____

☐   Gas cards   _____   _____

☐   New uniforms   _____   _____

☐   "Adopt" a needy family or children as an   _____   _____
office gift to the community.

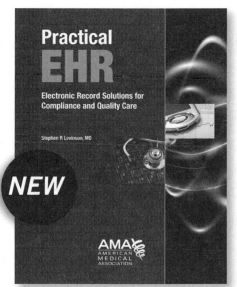
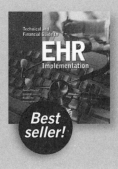
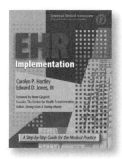
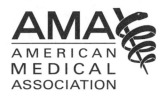

Online tool puts CPT® coding answers at your fingertips!

CPT® Network from the AMA provides expert answers and data fast—all from your desktop

Brought to you by the American Medical Association (AMA), *CPT® Network* is a subscription-based online inquiry system that helps you find fast, accurate answers to all of your coding questions—straight from the professionals who developed the Current Procedural Terminology (CPT®) code system.

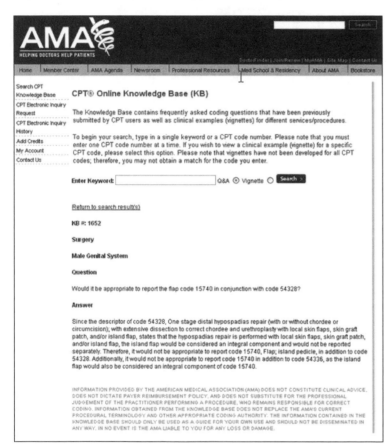

AMA member bonus: Six electronic inquiries and Knowledge Base access for one year free!

Quickly research the network's online Knowledge Base of commonly asked coding questions and clinical examples, as well as:

▫ Submit electronic inquiries directly to a CPT expert for timely, accurate results

▫ Track inquiry history

▫ Add credits to your account toward additional electronic inquiries (special pricing available)

▫ Easily update customer profile information

Subscribe today!

Call (800) 621-8335 to determine the subscription package that best meets your needs or visit ***www.cptnetwork.com*** for details.

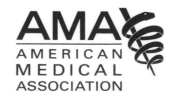
AMERICAN MEDICAL ASSOCIATION

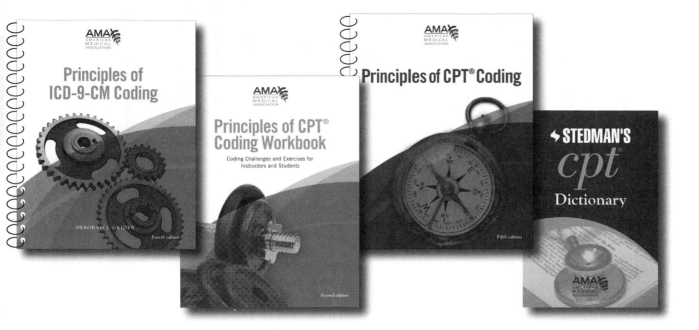

Principles of ICD-9-CM, fourth edition

This coding resource from the American Medical Association (AMA) provides helpful guidelines for identifying and locating the most appropriate codes for your practice and informative coding tips. Practical and educational, the fourth edition includes chapter learning objectives and checkpoint exercises, as well as a new timesaving CD-ROM teaching tool that lets instructors administer tests using AMA-developed questions and answers. New chapters cover symptoms, signs, ill-defined conditions, injury and poisoning, and an overview of ICD-9-CM, Volume 3, with a comparison to ICD-10-CM conventions.

Spiralbound, 8½" x 11", 356 pages, includes CD-ROM   ISBN: 978-1-57947-899-5

Principles of CPT® Coding Workbook, second edition

Newly revised and expanded, *Principles of CPT® Coding Workbook* provides in-depth instruction on key coding concepts, organized by Current Procedural Terminology (CPT®) code section. Extensive coding scenarios and operative procedure exercises accompany each chapter to test knowledge. The second edition features new chapters on Category II codes and appendixes found in the CPT codebook. This edition also contains new illustrations, decision-tree flowcharts and expanded chapters on E/M, medicine, surgery, anesthesiology and radiology.

Softbound, 8½" x 11", 300 pages   ISBN: 978-1-57947-883-4

Principles of CPT® Coding, fifth edition

Updated and revised by the AMA, this resource provides the most in-depth review available of the entire CPT codebook. Broad enough to educate the beginning coder while still offering relevant insight to those with more experience, the fifth edition explains the use of CPT codes and guidelines in a practical, easy-to-read style that addresses everyday coding challenges. Included are instructions on how to code from an operative report, and coding tips with hints on code assignments, bundling and payer policies.

Spiralbound, 8½" x 11", 580 pages   ISBN: 978-1-57947-967-1

Stedman's CPT® Dictionary

Understanding medical definitions can be one of the biggest struggles a coding or reimbursement professional faces. Developed by the AMA's CPT experts in conjunction with *Stedman's Medical Dictionary*, this resource makes coding easier by providing definitions of medical terms found within the CPT codebook descriptions.

Hardbound, 8" x 10", 425 pages   ISBN: 978-1-57947-882-7

For more information and to order online, visit *www.amabookstore.com* or call (800) 621-8335.

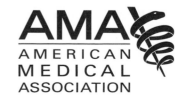

AMA
AMERICAN
MEDICAL
ASSOCIATION

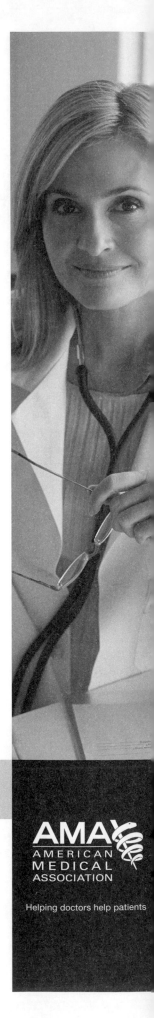